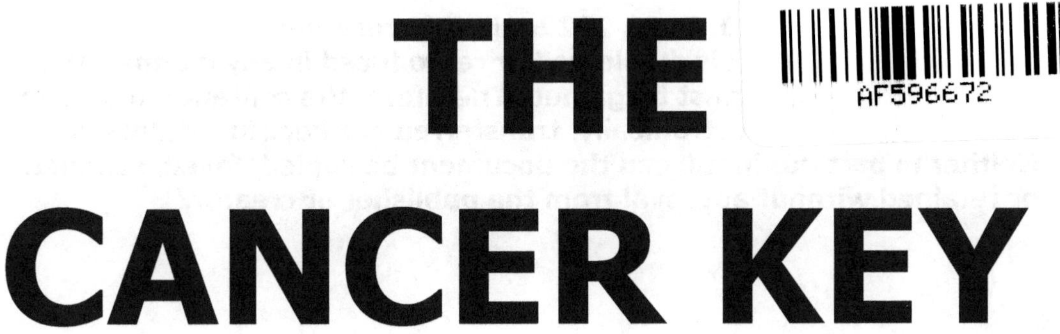

THE CANCER KEY

An Absolute New Understanding Of a Medical secret

By

Kendra J. Trask

TABLE OF CONTENT

CHAPTER FIVE

Introduction

Cancer is a sickness related to significant physical, close to home, social, and monetary repercussions for impacted people and their families. In a critical number of cases, the determination of cancer is either gone before by a time of progressive, vague side effects or found by routine screening, and people are then pushed into a hurricane of demonstrative testing, obtrusive methodology, and confounded medicines with next to no advance notice or potential chance to acclimatize their conditions. Much of the time, a multidisciplinary way to deal with therapy is fundamental, expecting patients to draw in with various clinical groups containing a few distinct claims to fame, frequently in various areas. Numerous patients have been moderately sounded proceeding the cancer occasion and in this manner are not refined purchasers of clinical benefits. Subsequently, it is an officeholder for medical services experts to have the option to work with patients' progress into care to limit their trouble and amplify their clinical results.

Challenges exist past the underlying determination and treatment period also. As per the National Cancer Institute (NCI), in excess of 12 million people in the United States are living with a background marked by cancer. More than half are living quite a ways past 5 years after the determination. Ladies contain a greater part of long-term survivors because of the positive results with bosom, cervical, and uterine cancers. The quantity of individuals living with a background marked by disease is projected to develop significantly over the course of the following 20 years for 2 significant reasons. In the first place, the quantity of Americans over age 65 is anticipated to be twofold between the years 2000 and 2030. Consequently, as a sickness fundamentally of more established grown-ups, cancer will likewise increment. Second, as the viability of cancer medicines improves, the number of patients restored from the infection will increment, and a significantly bigger rate will be living longer with the sickness while getting different "lines" of treatment (first-line, second-line, and so forth) after some time. The general interest in oncology administrations is supposed to increment by 48% by 2020, while the stockpile of oncologists will increment by just 14% in light of current patterns. These measurements highlight the requirement for a wide assortment of wellbeing experts and other help faculty to have an impact in empowering every single patient to get quality consideration that tends to all of their necessities all through the continuum of the sickness.

Inside this book, you will learn a lot of things associated with cancer and also useful tips and strategies to do while living with cancer.

CHAPTER ONE

The historical backdrop of cancer

The historical backdrop of cancer portrays the advancement of the area of oncology and its part throughout the entire existence of medication.

Early Diagnosis of Cancer
The earliest known depictions of cancer show up in a few papyri from Ancient Egypt. The Edwin Smith Papyrus was composed around 1600 BC (potentially a fragmentary duplicate of a text from 2500 BC) and contains a portrayal of cancer, as well as a methodology to eliminate bosom cancers by burning, wryly expressing that the infection has no therapy. Be that as it may, occurrences of cancer were interesting. In a concentrate by the University of Manchester, just a single case was found "in the examination of many Egyptian mummies, with few references to cancer in scholarly proof."
Hippocrates (c. 460 BC - c. 370 BC) portrayed a few sorts of cancer, alluding to them by the term karkinos (carcinos), the Greek word for crab or crawfish, as well as carcinoma. This comes from the presence of the cut surface of strong threatening growth, with "the veins extended on all sides as the creature the crab has its feet, whence it determines its name". Since it was against Greek practice to open the body, Hippocrates just portrayed and made drawings of ostensibly noticeable growths on the skin, nose, and bosoms. Treatment depended on the humor hypothesis of four organic liquids (dark and yellow bile, blood, and mucus). As indicated by the patient's humor, treatment comprised of diet, blood draining, and additionally intestinal medicines. Celsus (c. 25 BC - 50 AD) made an interpretation of karkinos into cancer, the Latin word for crab or crawfish.
In the second century AD, the Greek doctor Galen utilized oncos (Greek for enlarging) to portray all growths, holding Hippocrates' term carcinos for threatening cancers. Galen additionally utilized the postfix - oma to demonstrate carcinogenic injuries. It is from Galen's utilization that we determine the cutting-edge word oncology.
During that time it was found that cancer could happen in any place in the body, however, Hippocrates' humor- hypothesis-based treatment stayed well known until the nineteenth hundred years with the revelation of cells.
16th–19th century

A surgical operation to eliminate threatening Cancer
In the sixteenth and seventeenth hundred years, it turned out to be more satisfactory for specialists to take apart bodies to find the reason for death. The German teacher Wilhelm Fabry accepted that bosom cancer was brought about by milk coagulation in a mammary conduit. The Dutch teacher Francois de la Boe Sylvius, a supporter of Descartes, accepted that all infections were the result of synthetic cycles and that acidic lymph liquid was the reason for cancer. His contemporary Nicolaes Tulp accepted that cancer was a toxic substance that gradually spreads, and inferred that it was contagious.
The principal reason for cancer was distinguished by British specialist Percivall Pott, who found in 1775 that cancer of the scrotum was a typical sickness among chimney stack clears. Crafted by other individual doctors prompted different bits of knowledge, however when doctors began cooperating they could reach firmer determinations.

With the far-reaching utilization of the magnifying lens in the eighteenth hundred years, it was found that the 'cancer poison, in the long run, spreads from essential cancer through the lymph hubs to different destinations ("metastasis"). This perspective on the infection was first figured out by the English specialist Campbell De Morgan somewhere in the range of 1871 and 1874. The utilization of surgery to treat cancer had unfortunate outcomes because of issues with cleanliness. The prestigious Scottish specialist Alexander Monro saw just 2 bosom growth patients out of 60 enduring surgery for a considerable length of time. In the nineteenth hundred years, asepsis worked on careful cleanliness and as the endurance measurements went up, careful evacuation of the growth turned into the essential therapy for the disease. Except for William Coley who in the late nineteenth century felt that the pace of fix after surgery had been higher before asepsis (and who infused microscopic organisms into growths with blended results), disease therapy became reliant upon the singular specialty of the specialist at eliminating cancer. The fundamental reason for his outcomes may be that contamination invigorates the insusceptible framework to annihilate left cancer cells. During a similar period, the possibility that the body was comprised of different tissues that were comprised of millions of cells, laid rest the humor-speculations about substance irregular characteristics in the body.

Mechanism

The hereditary premise of cancer was perceived in 1902 by the German zoologist Theodor Boveri, teacher of zoology at Munich and later in Würzburg. He found a technique to produce cells with different duplicates of the centrosome, a construction he found and named. He hypothesized that chromosomes were unmistakable and communicated different legacy factors. He recommended that transformations of the chromosomes could produce a cell with limitless development potential which could be given to its relatives. He proposed the presence of cell cycle designated spots, cancer silencer qualities, and oncogenes. He hypothesized that cancers may be caused or advanced by radiation, physical or synthetic wounds, or pathogenic microorganisms.

Therapies

At the point when Marie Curie and Pierre Curie found radiation toward the finish of the nineteenth hundred years, they coincidentally found the principal successful non-careful cancer therapy. With radiation additionally came the principal indications of multi-disciplinary ways to deal with cancer therapy. The specialist was done working in disengagement however cooperated with emergency clinic radiologists to help patients. The entanglements in correspondence this brought, alongside the need of the patient's treatment in an emergency clinic office as opposed to at home, likewise made an equal course of gathering patient information into emergency clinic documents, which thusly prompted the principal measurable patient examinations.

The American Cancer Society was established in 1913 by 15 doctors and financial specialists in New York City under the name American Society for the Control of Cancer (ASCC). The ongoing name was embraced in 1945.

An establishing paper on cancer the study of disease transmission was crafted by Janet Lane-Claypon, who distributed a relative report in 1926 of 500 bosom cancer cases and 500 control patients of a similar foundation and way of life for the British Ministry of Health. Her earth-shattering work on cancer and the study of disease transmission was carried on by Richard Doll and Austin Bradford Hill, who distributed "Cellular breakdown in the lungs and Other Causes of

Death in Relation to Smoking. A Second Report on the Mortality of British Doctors" continued in 1956 (also called the British specialist's study). Richard Doll left the London Medical Research Center (MRC), to begin the Oxford unit for Cancer the study of disease transmission in 1968. With the utilization of PCs, the unit was quick to incorporate a lot of cancer information. Present-day epidemiological techniques are firmly connected to current [when?] ideas of infection and general wellbeing strategy. Throughout the course of recent years, extraordinary endeavors have been spent on social occasion information across clinical practice, emergency clinics, commonplace, state, and even country limits to concentrate on the relationship of ecological and social variables on cancer occurrence.
Cancer patient therapy and studies were confined to individual doctors' practices until World War II when clinical exploration communities found that there were enormous global contrasts in sickness occurrence. This understanding drove public general wellbeing bodies to empower the gathering of wellbeing information across practices and emergency clinics, a cycle tracked down in numerous nations today. The Japanese clinical local area saw that the bone marrow of casualties of the nuclear bombings of Hiroshima and Nagasaki was totally annihilated. They reasoned that unhealthy bone marrow could likewise be obliterated with radiation, and this prompted the improvement of bone marrow transfers for leukemia. Since World War II, patterns in cancer treatment are to enhance a miniature level the current treatment strategies, normalize them, and globalize them to track down fixes through the study of disease transmission and worldwide organizations.
In 1968 Michael A. Epstein, Bert Achong, and Yvonne Barr distinguished the principal human cancer infection, called the Epstein-Barr virus.

War on Cancer
The political 'battle' on cancer started with the National Cancer Act of 1971, a United States government law. The demonstration was expected "to correct the Public Health Service Act to reinforce the National Cancer Institute to all the more successfully complete the public exertion against disease". It was endorsed into regulation by then U.S. President Richard Nixon on December 23, 1971.
In 1973, cancer research prompted a virus war incident, where co-employable examples of revealed oncoviruses were found to be polluted by HeLa.
In 1984, Harald Zur Hausen found the first HPV16 and afterward HPV18 answerable for roughly 70% of cervical cancers. For revelation that human papillomaviruses (HPV) cause human cancer, Zur Hausen won a 2008 Nobel Prize.Beginning around 1971 the United States has contributed more than $200 billion to cancer research; that absolute incorporates cash contributed by open and confidential areas and establishments.
Notwithstanding this significant speculation, the nation has seen quite recently a five percent decline in the cancer passing rate (adapting to estimate and progress in years of the populace) somewhere in the range of 1950 and 2005. A longer future might be a contributing component to this, as cancer rates and death rates increment fundamentally with age, in excess of three out of five diseases are analyzed in individuals matured 65 and over.

What is Cancer?
Cancer is a gathering of in excess of 100 distinct sicknesses. It can foster any place in the body.

How Cancer Starts

Cells are the fundamental units that make up the human body. Cells develop and separate to make new cells as the body needs them. For the most part, cells kick the bucket when they go downhill or are harmed. Then, at that point, new cells have their spot.

Cancer starts when hereditary changes slow down this deliberate interaction. Cells begin to wildly develop. These phones might shape a mass called cancer. Growth can be carcinogenic or harmless. A carcinogenic growth is threatening, meaning it can develop and spread to different pieces of the body. A harmless growth implies the growth can develop however won't spread.

A few kinds of cancer don't shape cancer. These incorporate leukemias, most sorts of lymphoma, and myeloma.

Types of Cancer

Specialists partition cancer into types in light of where it starts. Four fundamental sorts of cancer are:

- **Carcinomas**. A carcinoma starts in the skin or the tissue that covers the outer layer of interior organs and organs. Carcinomas for the most part structure strong growths. They are the most widely recognized sort of cancer. Instances of carcinomas incorporate prostate cancer, bosom disease, cellular breakdown in the lungs, and colorectal cancer.
- **Sarcomas**. A sarcoma starts in the tissues that help and interface with the body. A sarcoma can foster in fat, muscles, nerves, ligaments, joints, veins, lymph vessels, ligaments, or bone.
- **Leukemia**. Leukemia is a cancer of the blood. Leukemia starts when solid platelets change and develop wildly. The 4 fundamental sorts of leukemia are intense lymphocytic leukemia, persistent lymphocytic leukemia, intense myeloid leukemia, and constant myeloid leukemia.
- **Lymphomas**. Lymphoma is cancer that starts in the lymphatic framework. The lymphatic framework is an organization of vessels and organs that assist with battling contamination. There are 2 fundamental kinds of lymphomas: Hodgkin lymphoma and non-Hodgkin lymphoma.

How Cancer Spreads

As carcinogenic growth develops, the circulation system or lymphatic framework might convey disease cells to different pieces of the body. During this interaction, the disease cells develop and may form into new growths. This is known as metastasis.

One of the principal puts cancer frequently spreads is to the lymph hubs. Lymph hubs are minuscule, bean-formed organs that assist with battling contamination. They are situated in bunches in various pieces of the body, like the neck, crotch region, and under the arms.

Cancer may likewise spread through the circulation system to far-off pieces of the body. These parts might incorporate the bones, liver, lungs, or cerebrum. Regardless of whether cancer spreads, it is as yet named for the area where it started. For instance, on the off chance that bosom cancer spreads to the lungs, it is called metastatic bosom disease, not cellular breakdown in the lungs.

Diagnosing Cancer

Frequently, a determination starts when an individual visits a specialist about a surprising side effect. The specialist will consult with the individual about their clinical history and side effects. Then, at that point, the specialist will do different tests to figure out the reason for these side effects.

Be that as it may, many individuals with cancer have no side effects. For these individuals, cancer is analyzed during a clinical trial for another issue or condition.

Some of the time a specialist finds cancer after a screening test in a generally solid individual. Instances of screening tests incorporate colonoscopy, mammography, and a Pap test. An individual might require more tests to affirm or invalidate the consequence of the screening test. For most cancers, a biopsy is the best way to make an unmistakable determination. A biopsy is the evacuation of a limited quantity of tissue for additional review. Get more familiar with making a determination after a biopsy.

CHAPTER TWO

Hereditary Changes and Cancer

Cancer is a hereditary infection — that is, the disease is made by specific changes in qualities that control the manner in which our cell's capability, particularly the way in which they develop and partition.

Qualities convey the guidelines to make proteins, which do a significant part of the work in our cells. Certain quality changes can make cells sidestep ordinary development controls and become cancer. For instance, some disease-causing quality changes increment the creation of a protein that makes cells develop. Others bring about the development of a distorted, and in this manner nonfunctional, type of protein that ordinarily fixes cell harm.

Hereditary changes that advance cancer can be acquired from our folks assuming the progressions are available in microorganism cells, which are the regenerative cells of the body (eggs and sperm). Such changes, called germline changes, are tracked down in each phone of posterity.

Cancer-causing hereditary changes can likewise be obtained during one's lifetime, as the consequence of blunders that happen as cells partition or from openness to cancer-causing substances that harm DNA, for example, certain synthetic compounds in tobacco smoke, and radiation, like bright beams from the sun. Hereditary changes that happen after origination are called substantial (or procured) changes.

There is a wide range of sorts of DNA changes. A few changes influence only one unit of DNA called a nucleotide. One nucleotide might be supplanted by another, or it could miss completely. Different changes include bigger stretches of DNA and may incorporate modifications, cancellations, or duplications of a significant length of DNA.

Some of the time the progressions are not in the genuine arrangement of DNA; for instance, the expansion or evacuation of substance marks, called epigenetic adjustments, on DNA can impact whether the quality is "communicated" — that is, whether and how much courier RNA is delivered. (Courier RNA thusly is meant to produce the proteins encoded by the DNA.)

As a general rule, cancer cells have more hereditary changes than ordinary cells. Be that as it may, every individual's cancer has a one-of-a-kind blend of hereditary modifications. A portion of these progressions might be the consequence of cancer, as opposed to the reason. As the disease keeps on developing, extra changes will happen. Indeed, even inside similar growth, disease cells might have different hereditary changes.

Hereditary Syndromes of Cancer

Acquired hereditary transformations assume a significant part in around 5 to 10 percent, everything being equal. Specialists have related transformations in unambiguous qualities with in excess of 50 genetic cancer conditions, which are messes that might incline people toward fostering specific diseases.

Hereditary tests for inherited cancer conditions can figure out if an individual from a family that gives indications of such a disorder has one of these transformations. These tests can likewise show whether relatives without clear infection have acquired a similar transformation as relative cancer-related change.

Numerous specialists suggest that hereditary testing for cancer risk be thought about when somebody has an individual or family ancestry that recommends an acquired disease risk

condition, as long as the experimental outcomes can be satisfactorily deciphered (that is, they can obviously tell whether a particular hereditary change is available or missing) and when the outcomes give data that will assist with directing an individual's future clinical consideration.
Cancers that are not brought about by acquired hereditary transformations can some of the time seem to "run in families." For instance, a common climate or way of life, for example, tobacco use, can make comparative diseases create among relatives. Notwithstanding, certain examples in a family —, for example, the kinds of cancer that create, other non-disease conditions that are seen, and the ages at which cancer creates — may recommend the presence of a genetic cancer disorder.

Regardless of whether cancer inclining transformation is available in a family, not every person who acquires the change will fundamentally foster disease.

Qualities involved in Genetic Cancer Conditions

• The most ordinarily transformed quality in all diseases is TP53, which delivers a protein that smothers the development of cancers. What's more, germline transformations in this quality can cause the Li-Fraumeni condition, an uncommon, acquired problem that prompts a higher gamble of fostering specific cancers.

• Acquired transformations in the BRCA1 and BRCA2 qualities are related to genetic bosom and ovarian cancer condition, which is a problem set apart by an expanded lifetime chance of bosom and ovarian diseases in ladies. A few different cancers have been related to this condition, including pancreatic and prostate diseases, as well as male bosom cancer.

• Another quality that delivers a protein that smothers the development of growth is PTEN. Transformations in this quality are related to Cowden condition, an acquired problem that expands the gamble of bosom, thyroid, endometrial, and different kinds of cancer.

Hereditary Tests for Hereditary Cancer Syndromes

Hereditary tests for transformations that cause inherited cancer conditions are typically mentioned by an individual's PCP or other medical services supplier. Hereditary directing can assist individuals with thinking about the dangers, advantages, and restrictions of hereditary testing in their specific circumstances.

A hereditary guide, specialist, or other medical services proficient prepared in hereditary qualities can assist an individual or family with understanding their experimental outcomes and making sense of the potential ramifications of test results for other relatives.

Individuals considering hereditary testing ought to comprehend that their outcomes might become known to others or associations that have genuine, legitimate admittance to their clinical records, for example, their insurance agency or business, on the off chance that their manager gives the patient's health care coverage as an advantage. Legitimate securities are set up to forestall hereditary segregation, including the Genetic Information Nondiscrimination Act of 2008 and the Privacy Rule of the Health Information Portability and Accountability Act of 1996.

Distinguishing Genetic Changes in Cancer

Lab tests called DNA sequencing tests can "read" DNA. By contrasting the arrangement of DNA in disease cells with that in typical cells, for example, blood or spit, researchers can distinguish hereditary changes in cancer cells that might be driving the development of a singular's cancer. This data might assist specialists with figuring out which treatments could work best against a specific growth.

Growth DNA sequencing can likewise uncover the presence of acquired transformations. To be sure, at times, the hereditary testing of growths has demonstrated the way that a patient's disease could be related to an inherited cancer condition that the family didn't know about.
Similarly, as with testing for explicit transformations in genetic cancer conditions, clinical DNA sequencing has suggestions that patients need to consider. For instance, they might advance unexpectedly about the presence of acquired transformations that might cause different sicknesses, in them or in their relatives.

CHAPTER THREE

MUTATION AND CANCER

Mutation of Cancer

Cancer is a consequence of the breakdown of the controls that manage cells. The reasons for the breakdown generally remember changes for significant qualities. These progressions are much of the time the aftereffect of transformations, changes in the DNA arrangement of chromosomes. Transformations can be tiny changes, influencing a couple of nucleotides or they can be exceptionally enormous, prompting significant changes in the construction of chromosomes. Both little and enormous mutations can influence the way of behaving of cells. Blends of transformations in significant qualities can prompt the advancement of cancer.

Mutation and Cancer

The strange ways of behaving exhibited by cancer cells are the consequence of a progression of mutation in key administrative qualities. The cells become continuously more unusual as additional qualities become harmed. Frequently, the qualities that are in charge of DNA fix become harmed themselves, delivering the phones significantly more defenseless to consistently expanding levels of hereditary pandemonium.

Liveliness that exhibit the connection between Chromosomes, Qualities and DNA

Most cancers are remembered to emerge from a solitary freak forerunner cell. As that cell partitions, the subsequent 'little girl' cells might procure various transformations and various ways of behaving throughout some undefined time frame. Those cells that gain a benefit in division or protection from cell passing will more often than not assume control over the populace. Along these lines, the cancer cells can acquire a large number of capacities that are not ordinarily found in the solid rendition of the cell type addressed.

Mutation in key administrative qualities (cancer silencers and proto-oncogenes) modifies the way of behaving of cells and might possibly prompt the unregulated development found in cancer.

For practically a wide range of cancer concentrated to date, maybe the progress from an ordinary, sound cell to a diseased cell is a stage-wise movement that requires numerous hereditary changes that amount to make the cancer cell. These transformations happen on the two oncogenes and cancer silencers. This is one motivation behind why cancer is substantially more predominant in more established people. To produce a cancer cell, a progression of transformations should happen in a similar cell. Since the probability of any quality becoming transformed is exceptionally low, it makes sense that the opportunity of a few distinct transformations occurring in a similar cell is genuinely far-fetched. Consequently, the cells in a 70-year-old body have had additional opportunity to collect the progressions expected to frame cancer cells however those in a youngster are substantially less liable to have obtained the imperative hereditary changes. Obviously, a few youngsters really do get cancer however it is significantly more considered normal in more established people.

In the lab, specialists have been endeavoring to make growth cells by modifying or presenting key administrative proteins. A few investigations have endeavored to characterize the insignificant number of hereditary changes expected to make a cancer cell, with fascinating outcomes.

In nature, transformations can aggregate in cells over the long haul and if the 'right' gathering of qualities is changed, cancer can result. A recent report showed that bone marrow foundational microorganisms in a sound individual collect numerous transformations as the individual ages. Only a couple of additional progressions to key qualities can cause cancer. The outcomes suggest that 'ordinary' cells and cancer cells may not be all that different generally speaking.

Inherited Mutations in Cancer

To convolute issues, obviously, the progressions expected to make a cancer cell can be achieved in a wide range of ways. Albeit all diseases need to conquer a similar range of administrative capabilities to develop and advance, the qualities included may contrast. Furthermore, the request in which the qualities become de-controlled or lost may likewise fluctuate. For instance, colon cancer cancers from two distinct people might include altogether different arrangements of growth silencers and oncogenes, despite the fact that the result (disease) is something very similar.

The extraordinary heterogeneity found in cancer, even those of similar organs, implies that determination and treatment are confounded. Current advances in the sub-atomic characterization of growths ought to permit the levelheaded plan of treatment conventions in light of the genuine qualities associated with some random case. New demonstrative tests might include the screening of hundreds or thousands of qualities to make a customized profile of cancer in a person. This data ought to consider the fitting of disease medicines outfitted to the individual hereditary changes that lead to unregulated cell development might be obtained in two distinct ways. It is conceivable that the transformation can happen progressively over various years, prompting the improvement of an 'inconsistent' instance of cancer. On the other hand, it is feasible to acquire useless qualities prompting the improvement of a familial type of a specific cancer type.

A few instances of cancers with realized inherited parts include:

• Breast cancer Inheritance of freak adaptations of the BRCA1 and BRCA2 qualities are realized gamble factors. Albeit many, while possibly not most, people with bosom cancer don't have distinguishable modifications in these qualities, having a freak structure improves the probability of creating bosom disease.

• Colon cancer Defects in DNA fix qualities, for example, MSH2 are known to incline people toward genetic non-polyposis colorectal disease (HNPCC).

• Retinoblastoma-Defects in the Rb growth silencer quality are known to cause this eye disease and a few different kinds of tumors. To a greater degree, this specific sickness can be tracked down in the segment on Rb

This is an inadequate rundown of the realized acquired cancer types, and it is sure that more acquired types of disease will be distinguished as the hereditary qualities of different sorts of cancer are explained.

Types of Mutation
The interaction by which proteins are made, and interpretation, depends on the 'perusing' of mRNA that was delivered by means of the course of the record. Any progressions to the DNA that encodes a quality will prompt a modification of the mRNA delivered. Thusly, the modified mRNA might prompt the development of a protein that no longer capabilities appropriately. In any event, changing a solitary nucleotide along the DNA of quality might prompt a totally non-utilitarian protein.
There are a few distinct ways DNA can be modified. The accompanying segment portrays the various types of hereditary change in more detail.

Point Mutations
Hereditary modifications can be put into two general classifications. The principal classification is contained changes that modify only one or a couple of nucleotides along a DNA strand. These kinds of changes are named point transformations.
At the point when ribosomes read a courier RNA particle, every three nucleotides are deciphered as one amino corrosive. These three-letter codes are called codons. To make a relationship to an English sentence: 'The heavy hitter ate the rodent' would contain 6 codons. The progressions brought about by transformation can prompt things like 'The fat bat ate the rodent.' or 'The fa' or 'The fat oca tat her at...' The effect on the protein relies upon where the change happens and the sort of progress.
The three-letter codons read by ribosomes might be changed by a mutation in one of three ways:

Nonsense mutation
The new codon makes the protein rashly end, delivering a protein that is abbreviated and frequently doesn't work as expected or by any stretch of the imagination.

Missense mutation
The new codon makes an inaccurate amino corrosive be embedded into the protein. The consequences for the capability of the protein rely upon what is embedded instead of the ordinary amino corrosive.

Frame-shift mutation
The misfortune or gain of 1 or 2 nucleotides causes the impacted codon and every one of the codons that follow to be misread. This prompts a totally different and frequently nonfunctional protein item.

Transcription Errors
Some DNA harm brings about a changed nucleotide or little gathering of nucleotides that can not be 'perused' by RNA polymerase. At the point when the RNA polymerase complex arrives at these spots, they will some of the time sidestep the harm by including nucleotides with an end goal to keep going, regardless of whether it implies placing in some unacceptable thing. This cycle is known as transcriptional mutagenesis and it might assume a critical part in the improvement of cancer.

Translocation
One more classification of transformations includes modifications of bigger measures of DNA, frequently at the level of the chromosome. These are called movements and include the breakage and development of chromosome sections. Frequently, breaks in two distinct chromosomes consider the development of two 'new' chromosomes, with new blends of qualities.

While it could create the impression that this wouldn't bring a lot of hardship, since every one of the qualities is as yet present, the cycle can prompt liberated cell development in various ways:
1. The qualities may not be deciphered and interpreted fittingly in their new area.
2. The development of quality can prompt an increment or a diminishing in its degree of record.
3. The breakage and rejoining may likewise happen inside a quality (as displayed in green above), prompting its inactivation.

For certain cancers, specific movements are exceptionally normal and may try and be utilized in diagnosing the sickness. Movements are normal in leukemias and lymphomas and have been less ordinarily distinguished in cancers of strong tissues. A model would be a trade between chromosomes 9 and 22 seen in more than 90% of patients with persistent myelogenous leukemia (CML). The trade prompts the development of an abbreviated type of chromosome 22 called the Philadelphia chromosome (after the area of its disclosure). This movement prompts the development of an oncogene from the abl proto-oncogene.

Different cancers that are frequently (or consistently) related to specific movements incorporate Burkitt's lymphoma, B-cell lymphomas, and a few kinds of leukemia.

Gene Amplification
In this exceptionally surprising cycle, the ordinary DNA replication process is genuinely defective. The outcome is that as opposed to making a solitary duplicate of a district of a chromosome, many duplicates are delivered. This prompts the development of many duplicates of the qualities that are situated on that district of the chromosome. Some of the time, such countless duplicates of the intensified district are delivered that they can really frame their own little pseudo-chromosomes called twofold moment chromosomes.

The gene on every one of the duplicates can be interpreted and made an interpretation of, prompting an overproduction of the mRNA and protein compared to the intensified qualities as displayed underneath. The squiggly lines address mRNA being delivered by means of the record of each duplicate of the quality.

While this cycle isn't found in ordinary cells, it happens frequently in cancer cells. On the off chance that an oncogene is remembered for the intensified district, the subsequent overexpression of that quality can prompt liberated cell development. Instances of this incorporate the enhancement of the Myc oncogene in a large number of growths and the intensification of the ErbB-2 or HER-2/neu oncogene in the bosom and ovarian diseases. On account of the HER-2/neu oncogene, clinical medicines have been intended to target cells overexpressing the protein item.

Gene enhancement additionally adds to quite possibly of the most concerning issue in cancer treatment: drug obstruction. Drug-safe cancers can proceed to develop and spread even within the sight of chemotherapy drugs. A quality ordinarily involved is called MDR for different medication obstructions. The protein result of this quality goes about as a siphon situated in the layer of cells. It is prepared to do specifically catapulting particles from the phone, including chemotherapy drugs. This evacuation delivers the medications insufficient.

Inversion, Duplications/ Deletions

Inversion

In these modifications, fragments of DNA are let out of a chromosome and afterward re-embedded on the contrary direction. As in the past models, this modification can prompt strange quality articulation, either by enacting an oncogene or de-initiating a growth silencer quality.

Duplications/Deletions

Through replication mistakes, a quality or gathering of qualities might be duplicated more than one time inside a chromosome. This is not quite the same as quality enhancement in that the qualities are not duplicated external to the chromosome and they are replicated an additional one time, as opposed to hundreds or thousands of times. Qualities may likewise be lost because of disappointment of the replication interaction or other hereditary harm.

Aneuploidy

Aneuploidy is the hereditary change that includes the misfortune or gain of whole chromosomes. Because of issues in the cell division process, the reproduced chromosomes may not separate into the little girl cells precisely. This can bring about cells that have an excessive number of chromosomes or a couple of chromosomes. An illustration of a genuinely normal aneuploidy condition that is irrelevant to cancer is Down disorder, in which there is an additional duplicate of chromosome 21 in every one of the cells of the impacted person.

In the liveliness underneath, duplicates of two chromosomes are made however when the cell partitions the chromosomes are not appropriated uniformly to the two cells that are shaped (little girl cells). The outcome is that one of the cells has an excessive number of chromosomes and one needs something more.

Cancer cells are all the time aneuploidy. People ordinarily have 46 chromosomes in their cells, however, cancer cells frequently have some more, some of the time more noteworthy than100. The presence of the additional chromosomes makes the cells temperamental and seriously disturbs the controls of cell division. There is at present a continuous discussion with respect to whether all cancers are aneuploidy. Whether or not that is the situation, obviously aneuploidy is a typical component of cancer cells.

Epigenetic Changes

Notwithstanding genuine modifications in DNA arrangement, quality articulation can be adjusted by changes to the DNA and chromatin that don't change the succession. Since these progressions don't adjust the arrangement of the DNA in the qualities, they are named epigenetic changes. Two kinds of epigenetic changes are portrayed underneath.

Methylation

In this modification, a few nucleotides in the DNA are changed by the expansion of a methyl (-CH3) gathering to the base. Methylation of DNA is related to the inactivation of that specific district of DNA. Unusual DNA methylation designs have been found in cancer cells. Like the progressions portrayed, methylation modifies the declaration of the impacted qualities.

Acetylation

In this epigenetic change, the histone proteins around which the DNA is wound become adjusted by the expansion of acetyl (- CH3CHO) gatherings. This modification prompts a slackening of the DNA: histone communication and is related to expanded quality articulation. The alteration of the cycles of expansion and evacuation of acetyl gatherings to DNA is a functioning area of cancer treatment research.

Causes of Mutation

As we have seen, cancer cells are made from ordinary forerunner cells by means of an aggregation of hereditary harm. The instruments by which the progressions are instigated have fluctuated. From an expansive perspective, the specialists of hereditary change (transformation) fall fundamentally into the classifications portrayed underneath and are examined top to bottom in the accompanying segment.

Spontaneous Mutations

Spontaneous mutation: The bases (A, T, G, and C) in DNA are modified or lost because of unrepaired replication blunders or irregular sub-atomic occasions. For instance, the deficiency of an amino gathering from cytosine, an ordinary base tracked down in DNA, prompts the development of uracil, a base not ordinarily tracked down in DNA. In the event that this change isn't distinguished and switched, a transformation can result. Once in a while, a whole base can be lost because of the cleavage of the connection between the DNA spine and the base. This prompts a hole in the DNA twofold helix, which, on the off chance that not fixed, can prompt a transformation whenever the DNA is replicated (for example during replication).

Induced Mutations

Induced mutation: Mutations can be initiated by uncovering organic entities (or cells) to different medicines. Probably the most widely recognized are:

Radiation-One of the principal known mutagens, radiation is a powerful inducer of transformations. Various sorts of radiation cause various kinds of hereditary changes. Bright (UV) radiation causes point transformations. X-beams can cause breaks in the DNA twofold helix and lead to movements, reversals, and different kinds of chromosome harm. Openness to the UV beams in daylight has been connected to skin cancer. Note that the DNA harming properties of radiation have been used in a few different radiation-based cancer therapies. Displayed underneath is a sort of transformation that is brought about by bright radiation. In this model, the barrage of the DNA twofold helix by UV beams makes two bases consolidate. This modifies the construction of the DNA and can prompt extremely durable changes in the event that not fixed.

One more kind of radiation is the energy transmitted by normally occurring radioactive components (like radon and uranium) or man-made sources like those found (and made) in atomic reactors. Radiation of this kind comes in various sorts and can make various sorts of harmful cells and tissues. Radiation can straightforwardly harm DNA or can cause the development of synthetic substances (for example responsive oxygen species or ROS) that can then harm DNA or other cell parts.

Openness to radiation from radioactive materials has been indisputably factual. Examinations of overcomers of the nuclear bombs dropped on Japan during World War II showed enormous expansions in leukemias not long after the openness and afterward increments in other cancer types over the accompanying decades.8

Hazardous measures of radioactive materials have additionally been unintentionally set free from thermal energy stations. Radiation openness because of the unintentional arrival of radioactive materials from the Chornobyl atomic reactor has been related to expansions in thyroid disease and other threatening cancers.9

Clinical imaging apparatus (like X-beam machines and CT scanners) additionally open patients to radiation. The sums utilized for any single test are not remembered to cause significant measures of cancer, however, the drawn-out effect of many tests over a time of years isn't clear.10 Likewise, the openness of plane travelers to full-body examines at air terminals isn't remembered to represent a gamble of cancer.11 Passengers flying in planes are additionally presented to radiation from space, yet at a low level and isn't remembered to represent a disease risk, in any event, for flight group members.

Chemical mutagens-Many various synthetic substances are known to cause transformations. These synthetic substances apply their impact by restricting DNA or the structure blocks of DNA and slowing down the replication or record processes. A few instances of powerful mutagens are benzo-a-pyrene, a substance found in tobacco smoke, and aflatoxin, a mutagen most frequently tracked down on inappropriately put away horticultural items.

Persistent aggravation of chronic irritation can prompt DNA harm because of the development of mutagenic synthetic substances by the cells of the insusceptible framework. A model would be the drawn-out aggravation brought about by contamination with the hepatitis infection.

Oxygen Radicals-During the catch of energy from food, which happens in our mitochondria, synthetic substances might be produced which are exceptionally responsive and are equipped for harming cell layers and DNA itself. These responsive oxygen intermediates (ROI) may likewise be produced by the openness of cells to radiation, as displayed underneath.

The mutagenic movement of ROI is related to the improvement of cancer as well as the exercises of a few anticancer therapies, including radiation and chemotherapy.

Abnormal Cell Division

During mitosis, it is conceivable that the phone division process neglects to partition the reproduced chromosomes precisely into two little girl cells. A blunder of this kind will prompt the development of aneuploid cells. The cells will either be missing or have acquired a critical number of qualities. This interesting system can make cells that are more inclined to unregulated cell division. As expressed beforehand, an enormous level of cancers disconnected from people is aneuploid.

In the event that a cell has a transformation in a quality whose protein item is liable for 'keeping an eye on the division cycle, things can quickly gain out of influence and the little girl cells of every division can turn out to be progressively strange.

Viruses as Mutagens

Infections are believed to be liable for a critical level of cancer cases. Infections can cause cancer in various ways and the way that each sort of infection works is probably going to be marginally unique. Some infections (counting numerous retroviruses) can cause transformations by embedding their qualities into the genome of the contaminated cell. The embedded DNA can annihilate or adjust the movement of impacted qualities.

Infections can likewise cause transformations in circuitous ways. For instance: Contamination with hepatitis infection can keep going for a long time. During that time the body's protection framework attempts to dispose of the infection by delivering poisonous synthetic substances. Those synthetic substances can make harm in any case sound 'spectator' cells, sending them not too far off that prompts cancer. There are various alternative ways that infections can cause cancer

Transposons as Mutagens

Transposons are short DNA arrangements that can move starting with one area in DNA and then onto the next area. Transposons encode a chemical, transposase, that demonstrates to graft the transposon into new areas in a genome (see schematic, underneath left, of a transposon) Transposons were found by Barbara McClintock and she won a Nobel prize for her work. The human genome contains many inactivated duplicates of transposons that have lost their capacity to move or 'leap' to new areas. Around half of the human genome is made out of 'dead' transposons.

The development of dynamic transposons can prompt transformations, alternating the movement of qualities. A noticeable illustration of transposon development (called rendering), is the shading of the portions in Indian corn (see underneath right). The transposons that are dynamic in people are believed to be associated with human sickness, including cancer.

CHAPTER FOUR

NUTRITION AND CANCER

Great nutrition is significant for Cancer patients.
Nutrition is a cycle wherein food is taken in and involved by the body for development, to keep the body sound, and to supplant tissue. Great nutrition is significant for good well-being. A sound eating routine incorporates food varieties and fluids that have significant supplements (nutrients, minerals, protein, starches, fat, and water) that the body needs.

Smart dieting propensities are significant during and after cancer treatment.
An eating routine with an emphasis on plant-based food varieties alongside customary activity will assist cancer patients with keeping a sound body weight, keeping up with strength, and diminishing incidental effects both during and after treatment.

An enlisted dietitian is a significant piece of the medical services group.
An enrolled dietitian (or nutritionist) is a piece of the group of well-being experts that assist with cancer treatment and recuperation. A dietitian will work with patients, their families, and the remainder of the clinical group to deal with the patient's eating regimen during and after cancer treatment.
Research has shown that remembering an enrolled dietitian for a patient's cancer care can help the patient live longer.

Cancer and cancer treatment might cause incidental effects that influence nutrition.
Nutrition issues are reasonable when growths include the head, neck, throat, stomach, digestion tracts, pancreas, or liver.
For some patients, the impacts of cancer treatment make it hard to eat well. Cancer treatments that influence nutrition include:
- Chemotherapy.
- Chemical treatment.
- Radiation treatment.
- Surgery.
- Immunotherapy.
- Stem cell transplant.

Cancer and cancer treatment might cause a lack of healthy sustenance.
Cancer and disease medicines might influence taste, smell, craving, and the capacity to eat sufficient food or assimilate the supplements from food. This can cause unhealthiness, which is a condition brought about by an absence of key supplements. Liquor misuse and corpulence might expand the gamble of lack of healthy sustenance.
Lack of healthy sustenance can make the patient powerless, tired, and incapable to battle contamination or finishing cancer treatment. Subsequently, a lack of healthy sustenance can diminish the patient's personal satisfaction and become hazardous. Lack of healthy sustenance might be exacerbated on the off chance that cancer develops or spreads.
Eating the perfect proportion of protein and calories is significant for recuperating, battling contamination, and having sufficient energy.

Anorexia and cachexia are normal reasons for the lack of healthy sustenance in cancer patients. Anorexia is the deficiency of craving or wants to eat. It is a typical side effect in patients with cancer. Anorexia might happen right off the bat in the sickness or later, on the off chance that cancer develops or spreads. A few patients as of now have anorexia when they are determined to have cancer. Most patients who have progressed cancer will have anorexia. Anorexia is the most widely recognized reason for the lack of healthy sustenance in cancer patients.

Cachexia is a condition set apart by shortcoming, weight reduction, and fat and muscle misfortune. Normally, patients with cancers influence eating and assimilation. It can happen in disease patients who are eating great but are not putting away fat and muscle as a result of growth development.

A few cancers fundamentally have an impact on the manner in which the body utilizes specific supplements. The body's utilization of protein, starches, and fat might change when growths are in the stomach, digestion tracts, or head and neck. A patient might appear to be eating enough, however, the body will most likely be unable to retain every one of the supplements from the food.

Cancer patients might have anorexia and cachexia simultaneously.

Impacts of Cancer Treatment on Nutrition

Central issues

• Chemotherapy and Hormone Therapy
. Chemotherapy and chemical treatment influence nutrition in various ways.
. Chemotherapy and chemical treatment cause different nutrition issues.
• Radiation Therapy
. Radiation treatment kills cells in the therapy region.
. Radiation treatment might influence nutrition.
• Surgery
. Surgery expands the body's requirement for supplements and energy.
. Surgery to the head, neck, throat, stomach, or digestion tracts might influence nutrition.
• Immunotherapy
. Immunotherapy might influence nutrition.
• Foundational microorganism Transplant
. Patients who get a stem cell transplant have extraordinary nutrition needs.

Chemotherapy and Hormone Therapy

Chemotherapy and chemical treatment influence nutrition in various ways.

Chemotherapy influences cells generally through the body. Chemotherapy utilizes medications to stop the development of cancer cells, either by killing the cells or by preventing them from partitioning. Sound cells that ordinarily develop and partition rapidly may likewise be killed. These remember cells for the mouth and gastrointestinal system.

The chemical treatment adds, blocks, or eliminates chemicals. It very well might be utilized to slow or stop the development of specific cancers. A few sorts of chemical treatments might cause weight gain.

Chemotherapy and chemical treatment cause different nutrition issues.

Incidental effects from chemotherapy might bring on some issues with eating and assimilation. At the point when more than one chemotherapy drug is given, each medication might cause different aftereffects or when medications cause a similar incidental effect, the incidental effect might be more serious.

The accompanying incidental effects that is normal:

- Loss of craving.
- Nausea.
- Regurgitating.
- Dry mouth.
- Bruises in the mouth or throat.
- Changes in the manner food tastes.
- Inconvenience gulping.
- Feeling full in the wake of eating a limited quantity of food.
- Obstruction.
- Looseness of the bowels.

Patients who get chemical treatment might require changes in their eating routine to forestall weight gain.

Radiation Therapy

Radiation treatment kills cancer cells and solid cells in the therapy region. How extreme the incidental effects rely upon the accompanying:

- The piece of the body that is dealt with.
- The absolute portion of radiation and the way things are given.

Radiation treatment might influence nutrition.

Radiation treatment to any piece of the stomach-related framework has incidental effects that cause nutrition issues. The vast majority of the incidental effects start a little while after radiation treatment starts and disappear half a month after it is done. A few incidental effects can go on for months or years after treatment closes.

The following includes the more normal incidental effects:

For radiation treatment to the cerebrum or head and neck

- Loss of craving.
- Nausea.
- Vomiting.
- Dry mouth or thick spit. The prescription might be given to treat a dry mouth.
- Sore mouth and gums.
- Changes in the manner food tastes.
- Trouble gulping.
- Pain while gulping.
- Being incapable to open the mouth completely.

For radiation treatment to the chest

- Loss of craving.
- Nausea.
- Vomiting.
- Trouble gulping.
- Pain while gulping.
- Choking or breathing issues brought about by changes in the upper throat.

For radiation treatment to the mid-region, pelvis, or rectum

- Nausea.
- Vomiting.
- Bowel impediment.
- Colitis.
- Diarrhea.
- Radiation treatment may likewise cause sluggishness, which can prompt a diminishing craving.

Surgery

Surgery expands the body's requirement for supplements and energy.

The body needs additional energy and supplements to recuperate wounds, battle contamination, and recuperate from surgery. On the off chance that the patient is malnourished before surgery, it might bring on some issues during recuperation, like unfortunate mending or contamination. For these patients, nutrition care might start before surgery.

Surgery to the head, neck, throat, stomach, or digestion tracts might influence nutrition.

Most cancer patients are treated with surgery. Surgery that eliminates all or some portions of specific organs can influence a patient's capacity to eat and process food.

The following are nutrition issues brought about by surgery:

- Loss of craving.
- Inconvenience biting.
- Inconvenience gulping.
- Feeling full in the wake of eating a limited quantity of food.

Immunotherapy

Immunotherapy might influence nutrition.

The symptoms of immunotherapy are different for every patient and the sort of immunotherapy drug given.

The accompanying nutrition issues are normal:

- Sluggishness.
- Fever.
- Nausea.
- Regurgitating.
- Looseness of the bowels.

Stem Cell Transplant

Patients who get a stem cell transplant have extraordinary nutrition needs.
Chemotherapy, radiation treatment, and different prescriptions utilized previously or during a stem cell transplant may cause incidental effects that hold a patient back from eating and processing food to the surprise of no one.

Normal incidental effects incorporate the accompanying:
• Mouth and throat injuries.
• Looseness of the bowels.
Patients who get a stem cell transplant have a high gamble of contamination. Chemotherapy or radiation treatment is given before the transfer to decline the number of white platelets, which battle contamination. These patients genuinely should find out about safe food take care and keep away from food varieties that might cause contamination.
After a stem cell transplant, patients are in danger of intense or persistent unit versus-have sickness (GVHD). GVHD might influence the gastrointestinal parcel or liver and change the patient's capacity to eat or assimilate supplements from food.

Nutrition Assessment in Cancer Care
• The medical services group might pose inquiries about diet and weight history.
• Directing and diet changes are made to work on the patient's nutrition.
• The objective of nutrition treatment for patients who have progressed cancer relies upon the general arrangement of care.

The medical services group might pose inquiries about diet and weight history.
Screening is utilized to search for medical conditions that influence the gamble of unfortunate nutrition. This can take care of find on the off chance that the patient is probably going to become malnourished, and assuming nutrition treatment is required.

The medical services group might pose inquiries about the accompanying:
• Weight changes over the course of the last year.
• Changes in the sum and kind of food eaten.
• Issues that have impacted eating, like loss of craving, nausea, regurgitating, looseness of the bowels, obstruction, mouth bruises, dry mouth, changes in taste and smell, or torment.
• Capacity to walk and do different exercises of day-to-day living (dressing, getting into or out of a bed or seat, cleaning up or showering, and utilizing the latrine).
An actual test is finished to really take a look at the body for general wellbeing and indications of infection. The patient is checked for indications of deficiency of weight, fat, and muscle, and for liquid development in the body.

Directing and diet changes are made to work on the patient's nutrition.
An enrolled dietitian can work with patients and their families to direct them on ways of working on the patient's nutrition. The enlisted dietitian gives care in light of the patient's nutrition and diet needs. Changes to the eating routine are made to assist with diminishing side effects from cancer or disease treatment. These progressions might be in the sorts and measures of food, how

frequently a patient eats, and how food is eaten (for instance, at a specific temperature or taken with a straw).
An enlisted dietitian works with different individuals from the medical services group to really take a look at the patient's nourishing wellbeing during cancer therapy and recuperation.
Notwithstanding the dietitian, the medical services group might incorporate the accompanying:
• Doctor.
• Nurture.
• Social specialist.
• Therapist.
The objective of nutrition treatment for patients who have progressed cancer relies upon the general arrangement of care.
The objective of nutrition treatment in patients with cutting-edge cancer is to provide patients with the most ideal personal satisfaction and control side effects that cause trouble.
Patients with cutting-edge cancer might be treated with anticancer treatment and palliative consideration, palliative consideration alone, or might be in hospice care. Nutrition objectives will be different for every patient. A few sorts of treatment might be halted on the off chance that they are not aiding the patient.
As the focal point of care goes from cancer treatment to hospice or end-of-life care, nutrition objectives might turn out to be less forceful, and a chance to mind intended to keep the patient as agreeable as could really be expected.

Treatment of Symptoms
• Anorexia
• Nausea
• Regurgitating
• Dry Mouth
• Sore Mouth
• Taste Changes
• Sore Throat and Trouble Swallowing
• Lactose Intolerance
• Weight Gain
At the point when symptoms of cancer or disease treatment influence typical eating, changes can be made to assist the patient with getting the supplements they need. Eating food varieties that are high in calories, protein, nutrients, and minerals are significant. Dinners ought to be wanted to meet the patient's nutrition needs and tastes in food.
Coming up next are a portion of the more normal side effects brought about by cancer and disease treatment and ways of treating or controlling them.

Anorexia
The next may assist cancer patients who with having anorexia (loss of craving or want to eat):
• Eat food varieties that are high in protein and calories. Coming up next are high-protein food decisions:
. Beans.
. Chicken.
. Fish.
. Meat.

. Yogurt.
. Eggs.
• Add additional protein and calories to food, for example, utilizing protein-strengthened milk.
• Eat high-protein food varieties first in your dinner when your craving is most grounded.
• Taste just limited quantities of fluids during dinners.
• Drink milkshakes, smoothies, squeezes, or soups on the off chance that you don't want to eat strong food varieties.
• Eat food varieties that smell wonderful.
• Attempt new food varieties and new recipes.
• Attempt blenderized drinks that are high in supplements (check with your primary care physician or enrolled dietitian first).
• Eat little dinners and sound snacks frequently over the course of the day.
• Eat bigger dinners when you feel great and are refreshed.
• Eat your biggest feast when you feel hungriest, whether at breakfast, lunch, or supper.
• Make and store limited quantities of most loved food varieties so they are prepared to eat when you are ravenous.
• Be pretty much as dynamic as conceivable so you will have a decent craving.
• Clean your teeth and flush your mouth to alleviate side effects and delayed flavor impressions.
• Converse with your primary care physician or enrolled dietitian in the event that you have eating issues like nausea, regurgitating, or changes in how food varieties taste and smell.
On the off chance that these eating regimen changes don't assist with anorexia, tube feedings might be required so you will get an adequate number of supplements every day.
Prescriptions might be given to increment craving.

Nausea
The next may assist cancer patients with controlling nausea:
• Pick food varieties that are an enticement for you. Try not to compel yourself to eat food that causes you to feel debilitated. Try not to eat your number one food variety, to abstain from connecting them to being debilitated.
• Eat food varieties that are tasteless, delicate, and simple to process, as opposed to weighty dinners.
• Eat dry food varieties, for example, saltines, breadsticks, or toast over the course of the day.
• Eat food varieties that are kind to your stomachs, like white toast, plain yogurt, and clear stock.
• Eat dry toast or saltines prior to getting up on the off chance that you have nausea in the first part of the day.
• Eat food varieties and drink fluids at room temperature (not excessively hot or excessively cold).
• Gradually taste fluids over the course of the day.
• Suck on hard confections, for example, peppermints or lemon drops on the off chance that your mouth has a terrible taste.
• Avoid food and drink serious areas of strength for with.
• Eat 5 or 6 little dinners consistently rather than 3 enormous feasts.
• Taste just limited quantities of fluid during dinners to abstain from feeling full or swelled.
• Try not to skip dinners and tidbits. An unfilled stomach might exacerbate your nausea.
• Flush your mouth when eating.

• Try not to eat in a room that has cooking smells or that is exceptionally warm. Keep the living space at an agreeable temperature and very much ventilated.
• Sit up or lie with your head raised for one hour in the wake of eating.
• Plan the best times for you to eat and drink.
• Loosen up before every cancer treatment.
• Wear garments that are free and agreeable.
• Track when you feel nausea and why.
• Consult with your primary care physician about utilizing anti-nausea medication.

Vomiting
The next may assist cancer patients with controlling vomiting:
• Try not to eat or drink anything until the vomiting stops.
• Drink limited quantities of clear fluids in the wake of vomiting stops.
• After you can drink clear fluids without regurgitating, drink fluids like stressed soups, or milkshakes that are kind to your stomach.
• Eat 5 or 6 little dinners consistently rather than 3 enormous feasts.
• Sit upstanding and twist forward in the wake of regurgitating.

Dry Mouth
The next may assist cancer patients with a dry mouth:
• Eat food varieties that are not difficult to swallow.
• Saturate food with sauce, sauce, or salad dressing.
• Eat food varieties and beverages that are exceptionally sweet or tart, like lemonade, to assist with making more spit.
• Bite gum or suck on hard sweets, ice pops, or ice chips.
• Taste water over the course of the day.
• Drink no kind of liquor, lager, or wine.
• Try not to eat food varieties that can hurt your mouth (like fiery, harsh, pungent, hard, or crunchy food varieties).
• Keep your lips sodden with lip demulcent.
• Flush your mouth each 1 to 2 hours. Try not to utilize mouthwash that contains liquor.
• Try not to utilize tobacco items and stay away from recycled smoke.
• Get some information about utilizing counterfeit spit or comparative items to cover, safeguard, and saturate your mouth and throat.

Sore Mouth
The accompanying can assist patients who with having mouth injuries:
• Eat delicate food varieties that are not difficult to bite, like milkshakes, fried eggs, and custards.
• Cook food varieties until delicate and delicate.
• Cut food into little pieces. Utilize a blender or food processor to make food smooth.
• Suck on ice chips to numb and alleviate your mouth.
• Eat food varieties cold or at room temperature. Hot food varieties can hurt your mouth.
• Drink with a straw to move fluid past the excruciating pieces of your mouth.
• Utilize a little spoon to assist you with taking more modest nibbles, which are simpler to bite.
• Avoid the accompanying:
. Citrus food varieties, like oranges, lemons, and limes.

. Spicy food varieties.
. Tomatoes and ketchup.
. Salty food varieties.
. Raw vegetables.
. Sharp and crunchy food varieties.
. Drinks with liquor.
• Try not to utilize tobacco items.
• Visit a dental specialist something like fourteen days prior to beginning immunotherapy, chemotherapy, or radiation treatment to the head and neck.
• Actually take a look at your mouth every day for injuries, white patches, or puffy and red regions.
• Flush your mouth 3 to 4 times each day. Blend ¼ teaspoon baking pop, ⅛ teaspoon salt, and 1 cup warm water for a mouth flush. Try not to utilize mouthwash that contains liquor.
• Try not to utilize toothpicks or other sharp articles.

Taste Changes
The next may assist cancer patients who with having taste changes:
• Eat poultry, fish, eggs, and cheddar rather than red meat.
• Add flavors and sauces to food varieties (marinate food varieties).
• Eat meat with something sweet, for example, cranberry sauce, jam, or fruit purée.
• Attempt tart food varieties and beverages.
• Use without sugar lemon drops, gum, or mints on the off chance that there is a metallic or unpleasant desire for your mouth.
• Utilize plastic utensils and don't drink straightforwardly from metal compartments on the off chance that food varieties have a metal taste.
• Attempt to eat your number one food variety, on the off chance that you are not disgusted. Attempt new food varieties while feeling your best.
• Find nonmeat, high-protein recipes in a veggie lover or Chinese cookbook.
• Bite food longer to permit more contact with taste buds, on the off chance that food tastes dull but not disagreeable.
• Keep food varieties and beverages covered, drink through a straw, turn a kitchen fan on while cooking, or cook outside on the off chance that scents irritate you.
• Clean your teeth and deal with your mouth. Visit your dental specialist for tests.

Sore Throat and Trouble Swallowing
The next may assist cancer patients who with experiencing an irritated throat or difficulty gulping:
• Eat delicate food varieties that are not difficult to bite and swallow, like milkshakes, fried eggs, oats, or other cooked cereals.
• Eat food varieties and beverages that are high in protein and calories.
• Saturate food with sauce, sauces, stock, or yogurt.
• Avoid the accompanying food varieties and beverages that can consume or scratch your throat:
. Hot food varieties and beverages.
. Spicy food varieties.
. Foods and juices that are high in corrosive.
. Sharp or crunchy food varieties.

. Drinks with liquor.
• Cook food varieties until delicate and delicate.
• Cut food into little pieces. Utilize a blender or food processor to make food smooth.
• Drink with a straw.
• Eat 5 or 6 little dinners consistently rather than 3 enormous feasts.
• Sit upstanding and twist your head somewhat forward when you eat or drink, and remain upstanding for somewhere around 30 minutes in the wake of eating.
• Try not to utilize tobacco.
• Converse with your primary care physician about tube feedings on the off chance that you can't eat to the point of serious areas of strength for remaining.

Lactose Intolerance

The next may assist patients who with having side effects of lactose narrow-mindedness:
• Use without lactose or low-lactose milk items. Most supermarkets convey food, (for example, milk and frozen yogurt) marked "lactose-free" or "low lactose."
• Pick milk items that are low in lactose, such as hard cheeses (like cheddar) and yogurt.
• Attempt items made with soy or rice, (for example, soy and rice milk and frozen pastries). These items don't contain lactose.
• Keep away from just the dairy items that give you issues. Eat little partitions of dairy items, like milk, yogurt, or cheddar, if possible.
• Attempt nondairy beverages and food varieties with calcium added.
• Eat calcium-rich vegetables, like broccoli and greens.
• Take lactase tablets while eating or drinking dairy items. Lactase separates lactose so it is more straightforward to process.
• Set up your own low-lactose or without lactose food varieties.

Weight Gain

The next may assist cancer patients with forestalling weight gain:
• Eat a lot of foods grown from the ground.
• Eat food varieties that are high in fiber, for example, entire grain bread, cereals, and pasta.
• Pick lean meats, for example, lean hamburgers, pork cut back of excess, and poultry (like chicken or turkey) without skin.
• Pick low-fat milk items.
• Eat less fat (eat just limited quantities of margarine, mayonnaise, pastries, and broiled food varieties).
• Cook with low-fat techniques, like searing, steaming, barbecuing, or simmering.
• Eat less salt.
• Eat food varieties that you appreciate so you feel fulfilled.
• Eat just when hungry. Think about directing or medication on the off chance that you eat as a result of pressure, dread, or discouragement. On the off chance that you eat in light of the fact that you are exhausted, find exercises you appreciate.
• Eat more modest measures of food at dinners.
• Work out day to day.
• Converse with your primary care physician prior to starting an eating regimen to get in shape.

Kinds of Nutritional Support

• Nutrition support helps patients who can't eat or process food regularly.
• Nutrition backing can be given in various ways.

Enteral Nutrition

• Enteral nutrition is additionally called tube taking care.

Parenteral Nutrition

. Parenteral nutrition conveys supplements straightforwardly into the circulatory system.
. The catheter might be put into a vein in the chest or in the arm.
Nutrition support helps patients who can't eat or process food typically.
It is ideal to take in food by mouth whenever the situation allows. A few patients will most likely be unable to take in sufficient food by mouth as a result of issues from cancer or disease treatment.
Nutrition backing can be given in various ways.
As well as directed by a dietitian, and changes to the eating regimen, nutrition treatment incorporates wholesome enhancement drinks and enteral and parenteral sustenance support.
Nourishing enhancement drinks assist cancer patients with getting the supplements they need. They give energy, protein, fat, starches, fiber, nutrients, and minerals. They are not intended to be the patient's just wellspring of nutrition.
A patient who can't take in the perfect proportion of calories and supplements by mouth might be taken care of utilizing the accompanying:
• Enteral nutrition: Nutrients are given through a cylinder embedded into the stomach or digestion tracts.
• Parenteral nutrition: Nutrients are implanted into the circulatory system.
Nutrition backing can further develop a patient's personal satisfaction during cancer treatment, however, may bring on some issues that ought to be considered prior to settle on the choice to utilize it. The patient and medical services group ought to talk about the damages and advantages of each kind of nutrition support. (See the Nutrition Needs at End of Life segment for more data on the utilization of nutrition support toward the finish of life.)

Enteral Nutrition

Enteral nutrition is additionally called tube taking care.
Enteral nutrition gives the patient supplements in fluid structure (equation) through a cylinder that is set into the stomach or small digestive system. The accompanying kinds of taking care of cylinders might be utilized:
• A nasogastric tube is embedded through the nose and down the throat into the stomach or small digestive system. This is utilized when enteral nutrition is just required for half a month.
• A gastrostomy tube is embedded into the stomach or a jejunostomy tube is embedded into the small digestive system through an opening made outwardly of the mid-region. This is typically utilized for long-haul enteral taking care or for patients who can't involve a cylinder in the nose and throat.
The kind of equation utilized depends on the particular requirements of the patient. There are equations for patients who have an extraordinary medical issue, like diabetes, or different requirements, like strict or social weight control plans.

Parenteral Nutrition
Parenteral nutrition conveys supplements straightforwardly into the circulation system. Parenteral nutrition is utilized when the patient can't take food by mouth or by enteral taking care of it. Parenteral taking care doesn't utilize the stomach or digestive organs to process food. Supplements are given to the patient straightforwardly into the blood, through a catheter embedded into a vein. These supplements incorporate proteins, fats, nutrients, and minerals. The catheter might be put into a vein in the chest or in the arm.
A focal venous access catheter is put underneath the skin and into an enormous vein in the upper chest. The catheter is set up by a specialist. This kind of catheter is utilized for long-haul parenteral taking care.
A fringe venous catheter is put into a vein in the arm. A fringe venous catheter is set up via prepared clinical staff. This kind of catheter is generally utilized for momentary parenteral taking care of patients who don't have a focal venous access catheter.
The patient is checked frequently for contamination or draining where the catheter enters the body.

Prescriptions to Treat Loss of Appetite and Weight Loss
• Medication might be given with nutrition treatment to treat loss of craving and weight reduction.
• Various sorts of medication might be utilized to treat loss of craving and weight reduction.
Medication might be given with nutrition treatment to treat loss of craving and weight reduction. Cancer side effects and aftereffects that influence genuinely should eating and cause weight reduction are dealt with ahead of schedule. Both nutrition treatment and medication can assist with diminishing the impacts that cancer and its treatment have on weight reduction.

Various kinds of medication might be utilized to treat loss of craving and weight reduction.
Prescriptions that further develop cravings and cause weight gains, like prednisone and megestrol, might be utilized to treat loss of hunger and weight reduction. Studies have shown that the impact of these prescriptions may not keep going long or there might be no impact. Treatment with a blend of prescriptions might work better compared to treatment with one medication. Patients who are treated with a blend of prescriptions might make more side impacts.

Nutrition Needs at End of Life
• Nutrition needs to change at end of life.
• Patients and families conclude how much nutrition and liquids will be given toward the finish of life.

Nutrition needs to change at end of life.
For patients toward the finish of life, the objectives of nutrition treatment are centered on alleviating side effects as opposed to getting an adequate number of supplements.

Normal side effects that can happen toward the finish of life incorporate the accompanying:
• Anorexia (loss of craving).
• Dry mouth.
• Gulping issues.

• Nausea.
• Regurgitating.

Patients who have issues gulping might find it more straightforward to swallow thick fluids than slender fluids.

Patients frequently don't feel a lot of yearning by any stretch of the imagination and may need next to no food. Tastes of water, ice chips, and mouth care can diminish thirst over the most recent couple of long stretches of life. Great correspondence with the medical services group is essential to comprehend the patient's progressions in nutrition needs.

Patients and families conclude how much nutrition and liquids will be given toward the finish of life.

Cancer patients and their parental figures reserve the privilege to settle on informed choices. The patient's strict and social inclinations might influence their choices. The medical services group might work with the patient's strict and social pioneers while simply deciding. The medical services group and an enrolled dietitian can make sense of the advantages and dangers of utilizing nutrition support for patients toward the finish of life. Generally speaking, there are a greater number of damages than benefits.

The dangers of nutrition support toward the finish of life incorporate the accompanying:

• Sepsis (microorganisms or their poisons in the blood or tissues) with the utilization of parenteral nutrition.
• Yearning (the unintentional taking in of food or liquid into the lungs) with the utilization of enteral nutrition.
• Injuries and breakdown of the skin where the enteral taking care of cylinder is embedded.
• Looseness of the bowels with the utilization of enteral and parenteral nutrition.
• Entanglements brought about by liquid over-burden (a condition where there is an excess of liquid in the blood) with the utilization of enteral and parenteral nutrition.

Nutrition Trends in Cancer

• Some cancer patients attempt extraordinary weight control plans to work on their visualization.
• Some cancer patients might take dietary enhancements.

Some cancer patients attempt extraordinary weight control plans to work on their visualization.

Cancer patients might attempt extraordinary weight control plans to make their therapy work better, keep incidental effects from therapy, or treat the actual disease. In any case, for the vast majority of these extraordinary weight control plans, there is no proof that shows they work.

Veggie lover or vegetarian diet

It isn't known whether following a veggie lover or vegetarian diet can assist with siding impacts from cancer treatment or the patient's visualization. On the off chance that the patient as of now follows a veggie lover or vegetarian diet, there is no proof that shows they ought to change to an alternate eating routine.

Macrobiotic eating routine
A macrobiotic eating routine is a high-starch, low-fat, plant-based diet. No investigations have shown that this diet will help cancer patients.

Ketogenic diet
A ketogenic diet limits starches and increments fat admission. The motivation behind the eating regimen is to diminish how much glucose (sugar) the growth cells can use to develop and duplicate. It is a hard eating routine to follow in light of the fact that definite measures of fats, starches, and proteins are required. Be that as it may, the eating regimen is protected.
A few clinical preliminaries are enrolling glioblastoma patients to concentrate on whether a ketogenic diet influences glioblastoma cancer movement. Patients with glioblastoma who need to begin a ketogenic diet ought to converse with their primary care physician and work with an enlisted dietitian. Be that as it may, it isn't yet known what the eating regimen will mean for the growth or its side effects.
Essentially, a review contrasting the ketogenic diet with a high-fiber, low-fat eating regimen in ladies with ovarian cancer or endometrial disease found that the ketogenic diet was protected and satisfactory. There isn't sufficient proof to know how the ketogenic diet will influence ovarian or endometrial growths or their side effects.

Some dietary enhancements by Cancer patients
A dietary enhancement is an item that is added to the eating regimen. It is generally taken by mouth, and for the most part, has at least one dietary fix. Cancer patients might take dietary enhancements to work on their side effects or treat their disease.

L-ascorbic acid (Vitamin C)
L-ascorbic acid is a supplement that the body needs in modest quantities to work and remain solid. It helps battle contamination, recuperate wounds, and keep tissues sound. L-ascorbic acid is tracked down in foods grown from the ground. It can likewise be taken as a dietary enhancement.

Probiotics
Probiotics are live microorganisms utilized as dietary enhancements to assist with absorption and ordinary entrail capability. They may likewise assist with keeping the gastrointestinal parcel sound.
Studies have demonstrated the way that taking probiotics during radiation treatment and chemotherapy can assist with forestalling looseness of the bowels brought about by those therapies. This is valid for patients who get radiation treatment in the mid-region. Cancer patients who are getting radiation treatment in the mid-region or chemotherapy that is known to cause looseness of the bowels might be helped by probiotics. Additionally, studies are seeing possible advantages of taking probiotics for cancer patients who are getting immunotherapy.

Melatonin
Melatonin is a chemical made by the pineal organ (minuscule organ close to the focal point of the cerebrum). Melatonin assists control the body's lay down with cycling. It can likewise be made in a research facility and taken as a dietary enhancement.

A few little investigations have shown that taking a melatonin supplement with chemotherapy or potentially radiation treatment for therapy of strong cancers might be useful. It might assist with diminishing symptoms of treatment. Melatonin doesn't seem to make side impacts.

Oral glutamine

Oral glutamine is an amino corrosive that is being read up for the therapy of looseness of the bowels and mucositis (aggravation of the covering of the stomach-related framework, frequently seen as mouth injuries) brought about by chemotherapy or radiation treatment. Oral glutamine might help forestall mucositis or make it less extreme.

Cancer patients who are getting radiation treatment to the midsection might profit from oral glutamine. Oral glutamine might decrease the seriousness of looseness of the bowels. This can assist the patients to go on with their treatment plan.

Hyperinsulinemia

Hyperinsulinemia is a condition wherein there are overabundance levels of insulin circling in the close family member to the degree of glucose. While it is frequently confused with diabetes or hyperglycemia, hyperinsulinemia can result from different metabolic sicknesses and conditions, as well as non-nutritive sugars in the eating regimen. While hyperinsulinemia is much of the time found in individuals with beginning phase type 2 diabetes mellitus, it isn't the reason for the condition and is just a single side effect of the sickness. Type 1 diabetes possibly happens when the pancreatic beta-cell capability is debilitated. Hyperinsulinemia should be visible in different circumstances including diabetes mellitus type 2, in youngsters, and in drug-actuated hyperinsulinemia. It can likewise happen in intrinsic hyperinsulinism, including nesidioblastosis. Hyperinsulinemia is related to hypertension, corpulence, dyslipidemia, insulin obstruction, and glucose narrow-mindedness. These circumstances are on the whole known as metabolic conditions. This nearby relationship between hyperinsulinemia and states of metabolic condition recommends related or normal instruments of pathogenicity. Hyperinsulinemia has been displayed to "assume a part in corpulent hypertension by expanding renal sodium maintenance". In type 2 diabetes, the cells of the body become impervious to the impacts of insulin as the receptors which tie to the chemical become less delicate to insulin fixations coming about in hyperinsulinemia and aggravations in insulin discharge. With a diminished reaction to insulin, the beta cells of the pancreas discharge expanding measures of insulin in light of the proceeded high blood glucose levels coming about in hyperinsulinemia. In insulin-safe tissues, a limited centralization of insulin is arrived at making the cells take up glucose and in this manner diminishing blood glucose levels. Studies have shown that the elevated degrees of insulin coming about because of insulin obstruction could improve insulin opposition.

Concentrates on mice with hereditarily diminished coursing insulin recommend that hyperinsulinemia assumes a causal part in high-fat eating routine prompted corpulence. In this review, mice with diminished insulin levels exhausted more energy and had fat cells that were reconstructed to consume some energy as intensity.

Hyperinsulinemia in youngsters can be the consequence of different ecological and hereditary variables. On the off chance that the mother of the newborn child is a diabetic and doesn't as expected control her blood glucose levels, the hyperglycemic maternal blood can establish a hyperglycemic climate in the hatchling. To make up for the expanded blood glucose levels, fetal pancreatic beta cells can go through hyperplasia. The quick division of beta cells brings about expanded degrees of insulin being discharged to make up for the high blood glucose levels.

Following birth, the hyperglycemic maternal blood is at this point not open to the youngster bringing about a quick drop in the infant's blood glucose levels. As insulin levels are as yet raised this might bring about hypoglycemia. To treat the condition, high fixation portions of glucose are given to the youngster as required to keep up with ordinary blood glucose levels. The hyperinsulinemia condition dies down following one to two days.

Symptoms and Signs

There are mostly no apparent side effects of hyperinsulinemia except if hypoglycemia (low glucose) is available. It is essential to take note that in certain individuals Insulin can be raised within the sight of ordinary glucose.

A few patients might encounter different side effects when hypoglycemia is available, including:

- Impermanent muscle shortcoming
- Cerebrum haze
- Exhaustion
- Nervousness
- Temporary thought disorder, or inability to concentrate
- Visual issues like obscured vision or twofold vision
- Cerebral pains
- Shaking/Trembling
- Thirst

On the off chance that an individual encounter any of these side effects, a visit to a certified clinical professional is encouraged, and demonstrative blood testing, for example, Fasting Insulin Levels, might be required.

Causes

Potential causes include:

- Neoplasm
- Starch mal-absorption
- Pancreatic cancer
- Polycystic ovary condition (PCOS)
- Trans fats

Since hyperinsulinemia and corpulence are so firmly connected it is difficult to decide if hyperinsulinemia causes stoutness or heftiness causes hyperinsulinemia or both.

Corpulence is portrayed by an overabundance of fat tissue - insulin expands the amalgamation of unsaturated fats from glucose, works with the passage of glucose into adipocytes, and restrains the breakdown of fat in adipocytes.

Then again, fat tissue is known to discharge different metabolites, chemicals, and cytokines that might assume a part in causing hyperinsulinemia. Explicitly cytokines discharged by fat tissue straightforwardly influence the insulin flagging outpouring and in this manner insulin emission.

Adiponectin is cytokines that are conversely connected with the percent muscle-to-fat ratio; that is individuals with a low muscle-to-fat ratio will have higher centralizations of adiponectin whereas individuals with a high muscle-to-fat ratio will have lower convergences of adiponectin.

In 2011, it was accounted for that hyperinsulinemia is unequivocally connected with low adiponectin fixations in corpulent individuals; however, whether low adiponectin plays a causal part in hyperinsulinemia still needs to be laid out.

- May prompt hypoglycemia or diabetes
- Expanded chance of PCOS
- Expanded amalgamation of VLDL (hypertriglyceridemia)
- Hypertension (insulin increments sodium maintenance by the renal tubules)
- Coronary Artery Disease (expanded insulin harms endothelial cells)
- Expanded chance of cardiovascular infection
- Weight gain and dormancy (potentially associated with an underactive thyroid)
- Corpulence and hyperinsulinemia have a few connections for certain kinds of cancer

Diagnosis

Fasting Insulin levels in the blood might be estimated as this can be raised within the sight of ordinary glucose. Diagnosis is frequently made by checking typical degrees of glucose that surpass 1.7 mmol/L (30 mg/dL) when 1 mg of glucagon is controlled IM or IV. Furthermore, pee tests or blood tests are additionally used to actually take a look at levels of ketones and low-free unsaturated fats.

After diagnosis, a great many people are expected to proceed with customary checkups for assessments.

Differential diagnosis

- Hyperinsulinemia is frequently confused with diabetes or hypoglycemia. These are independent, though related, conditions. Adipocytes will produce fatty substances within the sight of insulin; however, this alludes to a liver condition as opposed to a pancreatic one.

Treatment

Treatment is ordinarily accomplished by means of diet and exercise, in spite of the fact that metformin might be utilized to decrease insulin levels in certain patients (regularly where corpulence is available). A reference to a dietician is valuable. One more technique used to bring down unnecessarily high insulin levels is cinnamon, explicitly Ceylon cinnamon, as was exhibited when enhanced in clinical human preliminaries.

A sound eating regimen that is low in straightforward sugars and handled starches, and high in fiber, and vegetable protein is frequently suggested. This incorporates supplanting white bread with entire grain bread, diminishing admission of food varieties made fundamentally out of starch like potatoes, and expanding admission of vegetables and green vegetables, especially soy. Customary observing of weight, glucose, and insulin are encouraged, as hyperinsulinemia may form into diabetes mellitus type 2.

It has been displayed in many examinations that actual activity further develops insulin sensitivity.] The component of activity on further developing insulin responsiveness isn't surely known anyway thought practice makes the glucose receptor GLUT4 move to the layer. As more GLUT4 receptors are available on the layer more glucose is taken up into cells diminishing blood glucose levels which then, at that point, causes diminished insulin discharge and some mitigation of hyperinsulinemia.] Another proposed instrument of further developed insulin responsiveness by practice is through the AMPK movement. The valuable impact of the activity on hyperinsulinemia was displayed in a concentrate in 2009, where they found that further developing wellness through practice fundamentally diminishes blood insulin fixations. Besides, an eating regimen that comprises high measures of carbs has been connected to weight gain and corpulence in rodents. Albeit this has not been tried in people, it is expected that it could help with the counteraction of weight gain in people, and conceivably corpulence. Prescriptions have additionally been contemplated to treat hyperinsulinemia, albeit these could make a few side impacts, these could be utilized as another option.

Nutrient Sensing in Cancer

Cell-characteristic components of nutrient sensing are personally connected to versatile metabolic reactions, and these pathways assume basic parts in the mind-boggling and dynamic supplement climate of developing cancer. Supplement responsive record factors (e.g., HIF, SREBP, ATF4) and flagging pathways (e.g., mTORC1, AMPK) permit growth cells to tune their metabolic result and methodologies to vacillations in nutrient accessibility, in this manner adjusting cancer cell multiplication and endurance with a blend of anabolic and versatile reactions. Coupling these supplement detecting instruments to the control of reusing and rummaging processes, for example, autophagy and macropinocytosis, further upgrades the flexibility of supplements inside growths. Here, we talk about the key supplement detecting pathways dynamic in disease cells, how oncogenic occasions impact these pathways and their reasonable commitments to cancer development and endurance. A superior comprehension of supplement detecting methodologies and metabolic transformations inside the growth microenvironment is basic to characterizing and focusing on metabolic weaknesses in disease. Cancer cells can flourish in supplement denied conditions, conveying explicit transformations that empower them to utilize unconventional techniques for supplement procurement. They have the limit of finely observing the open extraneous supplements, whose accessibility wavers all through various oncogenesis stages, to coordinate suitable metabolic reactions. The capability of cancer cells in these cycles might be accomplished by the enlistment of quality articulation programs that regulate the movement of supplement carriers and explicit metabolic catalysts. They have the limit of finely observing the open extraneous supplements, whose accessibility wavers all through various oncogenesis stages, to coordinate suitable metabolic reactions. The capability of cancer cells in these cycles might be accomplished by acceptance of quality articulation programs that regulate the movement of supplement carriers and explicit metabolic chemicals [9]. For example, hypoxia sets off the declaration of record factors, called hypoxia-inducible variables (HIF), which invigorate glucose take-up, lactate commodity, glycolysis, and angiogenesis.

The capability of cancer cells in these cycles might be accomplished by the enlistment of quality articulation programs that regulate the movement of supplement carriers and explicit metabolic compounds. For example, hypoxia sets off the declaration of record factors, called hypoxia-inducible variables (HIF), which invigorate glucose take-up, lactate commodity, glycolysis, and angiogenesis. Besides, cholesterol consumption instigates initiation of sterol administrative component restricting proteins (SREBP), a group of record factors that invigorate the statement of pretty much each and every catalyst expected for once more combination of unsaturated fat and sterol lipids, likewise prompting increased low-thickness lipoprotein (LDL) receptor articulation and improved NADPH creation.

Outstandingly, most cancer drug testing has been finished in 2D societies. Be that as it may, 3D cancer cell models are proposed as further developed models for starting medication screening, in light of their capacity to demonstrate cell communications and regular supplement slopes happening in a connective or ineffectively vascularized cancer microenvironment.

Levels of both glucose and lactate are fundamental for the endurance of cancer cells in three-layered settings; in this manner, the carriers controlling these are worth further examination [39]. Notwithstanding the extracellular degrees of glucose estimated at 1 mM, we construe that the glucose might be depleted in the center of the spheroid because of regular slopes and dissemination, true to form in such a model. This in addition to an accepted low oxygen fractional tension in the spheroid center might be driving putrefaction and connected with the metabolic changes seen here.

Flagging Pathways Involved in Nutrient Sensing Control in Cancer Stem Cells:

The last option incorporate caloric limitation or glucose hardship, which diminishes Warburg-type breath and temper insulin and additionally insulin-like development factor flagging. The resulting changes in the miniature ecological supplement supply can affect cancer cell flagging pathways, development, and chemotherapeutic responsiveness.
It further gives 3-phosphoglycerate to serine, glycine, and purine nucleotide biosynthesis and pyruvate, which outfits alanine and other amino acids and the anaplerotic TCA cycle substrate oxaloacetate. Additionally, glutaminolysis is an anaplerotic wellspring of α-ketoglutarate, another TCA cycle middle of the road, that provisions aspartate and asparagine as well as citrate by means of reductive carboxylation. At long last, the neomorphic movement of isocitrate dehydrogenase (IDH) missense freaks produces the novel oncometabolite 2-hydroxyglutarate, which keeps up with the undifferentiated condition of the impact cell populace in intense myelogenous leukemia.
Cancer cells distinctively have a high multiplication rate. Since cancer development relies upon energy-consuming anabolic cycles, including biosynthesis of protein, lipid, and nucleotides, numerous cancer-related conditions, including discontinuous oxygen lack because of inadequate vascularization, oxidative pressure, and supplement hardship, result from quick development. To adapt to these ecological stressors, cancer cells, including disease foundational microorganisms, should adjust their digestion to keep up with cell homeostasis. It is notable that cancer foundational microorganisms (CSC) reconstruct their digestion to adjust to living in hypoxic specialties. They for the most part change from oxidative phosphorylation to expanded high-impact glycolysis even within the sight of oxygen. Be that as it may, rather than most separated cancer cells depending on glycolysis, CSCs can be exceptionally glycolytic or oxidative phosphorylation-subordinate, showing high metabolic versatility. Albeit the impact of the metabolic and supplement detecting pathways on the support of stemness has been perceived, the sub-atomic instruments that interface these pathways to stemness are not notable. Here in this survey, we portray the most significant flagging pathways associated with supplement detecting and cancer cell endurance. Among them, Adenosine monophosphate (AMP)- actuated protein kinase (AMPK) pathway, mTOR pathway, and Hexosamine Biosynthetic Pathway (HBP) are basic sensors of cell energy and supplement status in cancer cells and communicate in mind-boggling and dynamic ways.
Growths are not uniform yet rather heterogeneous in capability. The contribution of foundational microorganism cancer (CSC) subpopulations has been exhibited in practically all human diseases. These cells have the ability to reproduce the whole growth and are frequently signified as cancer-starting cells (TICs). They likewise drive growth development, metastatic spread, and backslide, making them an overwhelming yet encouraging objective to dispense with the disease.

Cancer cells reconstruct their metabolic methodology to address their issues, for example, their high multiplication rate: they instigate quick ATP age to keep up with energy status, increment the biosynthesis of macromolecules, and initiate severe guidelines of the cell redox status. Non-threatening cells acquire ATP, an energy source fundamental for endurance, from both glycolysis and mitochondrial oxidative phosphorylation (OXPHOS). Conversely, cancer cells for the most part get ATP from glycolysis as opposed to OXPHOS, even within the sight of satisfactory oxygen fixation (Warburg impact). More or less, most cancer cells rely upon glycolysis to produce ATP, in any event, when oxygen is free.

In contrast with glycolysis-based separated mass growth cells, CSCs display high versatility showing an unmistakable metabolic aggregate that can change their digestion to miniature ecological changes relying upon the kind of disease by helpfully moving energy yield starting with one pathway then onto the next or getting middle of the road metabolic aggregates. Regardless, the mitochondria's capability is significant and centers around CSC usefulness. As well as being a critical wellspring of ATP for cells, mitochondria are engaged with the guideline of many flagging pathways in CSCs, for example, mitochondrial unsaturated fat oxidation (FAO) for the age of ATP and NADPH.

No matter what the essential metabolic aggregate in individual cells, mitochondria frequently will more often than not control stemness properties. Expanded mitochondrial biogenesis and mass perceive cells with improved self-reestablishment capacity and chemoresistance, independent of the kind of cancer. Foundational microorganism mitochondria are more modest in number and show diminished movement compared with separated cells. This large number of attributes brings about diminished ROS levels in foundational microorganisms. The evident reliance of CSCs, independent of their essential metabolic aggregate on mitochondrial capability, is a formerly unnoticed Achilles' heel modifiable for restorative purposes.

The multiplication of cancer cells to a great extent relies upon their nourishing environmental elements, particularly the accessibility of glucose. It is notable that CSCs get a significant measure of their energy by means of vigorous glycolysis, which is quicker than OXPHOS and undeniably less productive to create ATP per unit of glucose consumed, inciting a strangely high pace of glucose take-up. In CSCs, glutamine is additionally effectively assimilated. Albeit the commitment of the metabolic and supplement detecting pathways to stemness conservation has been illustrated, the sub-atomic instruments interfacing stemness with the supplement detecting courses are not surely known. Be that as it may, among these pathways, mTOR and AMPK pathways' commitment, along with the hexosamine biosynthesis pathway (HBP), is perhaps the most critical.

The metabolic aggregate of CSCs has been the focal point of broad concentrate as of late. It is essential to accentuate that growths show cell heterogeneity. While CSCs favor glycolysis and have fewer mitochondria, they have high metabolic flexibility that permits them to flourish in states of supplement and stress miniature ecological vacillations. Utilizing supplement detecting pathways, for example, HBP and those controlled by mTOR and AMPK, foundational microorganisms support energy yield by restraining fundamental cycles like OXPHOS and improving others like glycolysis. In the resulting segments, we will make sense of how HBP is controlled by the admission of supplements like fats, amino acids, and nucleic acids, changing over it into a significant supplement sensor for these particles' varieties. All the more in this way, we will portray how the mammalian objective of rapamycin (mTOR) and AMP-enacted protein kinase (AMPK) pathways take part in supplement detecting as an approach to controlling cell movement. We will likewise portray how the collaboration among these pathways changes the cell reaction to supplements and is fundamental for stemness support. Albeit metabolic reconstructing is a quality of self-reestablishing cancer foundational microorganisms, very little is had some significant awareness of how their digestion is directed to control CSC aggregate. In such a manner, it has been exhibited that the restraint of the HBP-Hypoxia inducible component 1 (HIF-1α) pivot repeals glycolysis improvement and diminishes the CSC-like subpopulation. Hypoxia-inducible variables (HIFs) are ace record factors controlling the transformation of disease cells to hypoxic conditions frequently produced in cancers as an outcome of quick development. Significantly, it has been exhibited that HIFs control different periods of tumorigenesis and are ordinarily connected in cancer cells with changes in metabolic reconstructing. Surprisingly, it has been shown that O-GlcNAcylation controls cancer digestion and endurance stress announcing controlling the HIF-1α flagging pathway. In such a manner, we have laid out that O-GlcNAc and the movement of OGT are personally connected with the cell's nourishing status, as recently announced in a few cell frameworks. Prominently, we additionally found that expanded O-GlcNAc levels appear to be essential for an endogenous pressure reaction related to cancer cell endurance. In accordance with this, our discoveries have confirmed that starvation improves the declaration of foundational microorganism markers. In any case, significantly, it approves the discernment that the OGT movement and HBP pathway are firmly coordinated with the nourishing status of the cells and adds to the guideline of stemness support.

CHAPTER FIVE

Treatment implication

Cancer prevention and screening

An essential method of cancer prevention and early identification in the United States is the far and wide act of screening. Albeit numerous methodologies for early identification and counteraction are accessible, antagonistic results, for example, over-diagnosis and overtreatment are predominant among those using these methodologies. Expansive utilization of mammography and prostate cancer screening are key models representing the potential damages originating from the identification of lethargic injuries and the resulting overtreatment. Moreover, there are a few cancers for which counteraction methodologies don't at present exist. Clinical and exploratory proof has extended how we might interpret cancer commencement and movement, and have educated the advancement of improved, exact methods of disease counteraction and early identification. Ongoing cancer counteraction and early identification developments have started moving towards the reconciliation of sub-atomic information and hazard delineation profiles to take into consideration a more precise portrayal of in-danger people. The eventual fate of cancer counteraction and early identification endeavors ought to accentuate the consolidation of accuracy disease anticipation reconciliation where screening and cancer avoidance regimens can be matched to one's gamble of cancer due to known genomic and ecological variables.

Many years of fundamental natural and clinical examination have lain out that a long hatching time is expected for the improvement of threatening injuries. Indeed, even after openness to referred to cancer-causing agents, like tobacco or human papilloma infection (HPV), cancers call for significant investment to develop.1 Therefore, there is enough of a chance to distinguish early precancerous injuries and intercede during the commencement and advancement steps of the cancer-causing process, in this manner switching or postponing the course of disease movement by means of screening and counteraction. The genomic transformation and mechanical advances are drivers in translating the sub-atomic occasions adding to sickness movement and making accuracy focusing on cancer evaluation and counteraction inside the domain of utilization for the advantage of high-risk people and afterward, hopefully, everybody. In this survey, we will zero in on the ongoing utility of accuracy cancer counteraction and screening methodologies, as well as examine propels empowering our capacity to diminish over diagnosis of sores that may not conclusively progress to disease and distinguish ways to deal with recognize extra underdiagnosed injuries with a high opportunity of movement to cancer.

The role of Cancer prevention and early identification

Cancer is a main source of death in the United States, second just to coronary illness. In 2018, it is assessed that ~1.7 million cancers will be analyzed in people, with a comparing 609,000 disease-related passing. Every year, the quantity of occurrence cancer cases keeps on expanding all around the world. By 2020, the quantity of occurrence cancer cases analyzed every year is supposed to ascend to 15 million. Luckily, a few disease types, specifically colorectal, bosom, and prostate cancer, can be distinguished by routine screening which prompts the early identification of threatening injuries.

Prevention is defined as "the protection of health by personal and community-wide efforts''. These endeavors are accomplished by portraying the weight of cancer, distinguishing its causes, and assessing and carrying out disease counteraction intercessions. Verifiable points of view of cancer counteraction research have fundamentally centered on diminishing occurrence and disease-related mortality. Early endeavors in cancer counteraction zeroed in on both orchestrated synthetic substances (for example retinoid, tamoxifen, and so forth) and regular mixtures (for example β-carotene, omega-3 fish oil, and so forth.). Endeavors have all the more as of late expanded to incorporate intercessions zeroed in on 'pre-sickness' or those expected to postpone carcinogenesis. These undertakings, be that as it may, are easy to talk about, but not so easy to do. Public and worldwide level associations, for example, the National Cancer Institute (NCI), the World Health Organization (WHO), and the International Agency for Research on Cancer (IARC) have the assets and capacities to precisely address the populace level weight of cancer. Notwithstanding, counteraction drives ought to initially significantly affect the individual level to eventually mean a populace level advantage, suggesting the view that populace wellbeing is the aggregate wellbeing experience of people.

Cancer risk is impacted by a combination of hereditary and ecological variables, for example, conduct, way of life, and natural openings. A people's gamble is the amount of these different variables however, the impact greatness of a solitary component is challenging to evaluate. In vitro and in vivo exploratory examination has considered the distinguishing proof of qualities, like FOXA2, PIK3CA, and RB1, which can drive cancer commencement and movement. This interaction turns out to be more mind-boggling with the expansion of new hereditary occasions. These confounded hereditary marks might be additionally impacted by ecological openings. Populace inferable division (PAF) is an estimation expected to be all the more likely to characterize the infection hazard of an individual ecological openness. For instance, a review directed in the United Kingdom assessed a PAF of 19.4% for tobacco and 3.7% for word-related openings, adding to ~60,800 and 11,500 cancer cases every year, separately. Be that as it may, different variables related to one's gamble of cancer, for example, time allotment uncovered, openness level, and openness aggregate, are not represented in this computation. In this manner, deciding the genuine effect of individual variables on one's general cancer risk is hazardous to determine.

A few counteractions and early identification components have been distinguished to help with diminishing cancer occurrence and are staggered, including essential, optional, and tertiary cycles. Essential cancer counteraction includes the immediate aversion or decrease in openness to known cancer-causing factors.6 Key instances of essential anticipation incorporate tobacco discontinuance, changes in diet (for example diminished red meat utilization, restricting greasy food varieties), and expanded actual work. Essential counteraction techniques include adjusting way of life factors that present a gamble of creating cancer (e.g., work out, tobacco discontinuance, and nourishing enhancements) and defensive therapeutics (for example immunization) which have exhibited long-haul viability for cancer counteraction. Auxiliary counteraction assists with deteriorating, restraining or turning around carcinogenesis. These strategies frequently include the early identification, therapy, or evacuation of precancerous sores, which will be additionally characterized in the following segment. For instance, colorectal adenomas or beginning phase colorectal cancers can be distinguished through screening by colonoscopy, an optional counteraction methodology. Furthermore, testing for HPV DNA or co-testing with the cytology-based Pap smear can distinguish cervical cancer-related HPV diseases. Tertiary counteraction can be started after a determination of cancer to work on personal satisfaction and survivorship. It is essential to take note that the meanings of essential, auxiliary, and tertiary counteraction can fluctuate, but the general message of anticipation is something very similar. Monitoring the intricacies of individual and populace cancer risk and being furnished with a large number of counteraction methodologies places the medical services local area in an excellent situation for disease counteraction.

The case for the early identification of Cancer

Multistep tumorigenesis is expected for the change of an ordinary cell to a carcinogenic cell. Boland and Ricardo give an improved model of tumorigenesis: an organic entity collects various hereditary transformations because of openings or blunders during DNA combination or mitosis, which prompts the distorted development of a phone through a progression of shortening or missense changes and hereditary cancellations. However most mistakes happening during replication are quiet, nonfunctional, rectified, or bring about cell passing, once in a while, a quality becomes transformed, fundamentally through a blend of frame shifts (inclusion/cancellations) and missense transformations that influence the usefulness of the phone. Progressive substantial genomic or epigenomic modifications might give extra cell benefits that lead to intrusive cancer. Information from a far-reaching assessment of sub-atomic disease subtypes demonstrated that 5-10 hereditary modifications are expected to instigate a threatening aggregate. Concentrates on colorectal cancer have exhibited that somewhere around seven hereditary occasions are fundamental for change. In a few genetic and irregular cancers, genomic precariousness seems to happen in the early disease stages with moderate destabilization over the long haul.

Frequently the pathways adjusted during early cancer advancement influence explicit physiological cycles, for example, tissue fix, wound recuperating, vascularization, or the co-choice of encompassing cells through direct contact, discharged development variables, or quality exchange by extracellular vesicle emission. The substantial transformation hypothesis recommends that stochastic physical changes bring about the determination of hereditary modifications that give benefit uncontrolled multiplication and tumorigenesis. Be that as it may, this hypothesis has not been experimentally tried and has a few deficiencies, including no notice of strategies that can instigate DNA modifications without transformation, for example, epigenetic changes, or the consideration of the growth microenvironment (the impact of the stroma and insusceptible milieu). Exploratory proof has recommended that either worldwide hereditary precariousness, for example, chromosomal or microsatellite unsteadiness from issues during the cell cycle or DNA fix (e.g., crisscross fix) inadequacy is required for the movement of most cancer. The 'helpful' tissue microenvironment prompted by the cancer cells or as a component of a premalignant specialty is fundamental for cancer development and results in distinguishable changes in the tissue. Models of pancreatic disease have exhibited the need for fibroblasts in cancer cell proliferation, while extra carcinogenesis models have shown that enlistment of endothelial cells to the growth is fundamental for development past 1-2 mm3. Cancer advances in spatial and transient spaces, where it might require a very long time to a very long time for typical cells to progress into obtrusive diseases; furthermore, different cell clones inside an individual or inside a similar cancer type in others can developmentally wander to present as discrete substances. Subsequently, the sub-atomic abnormalities that at first lead to change proceed with their advancement and further form into heterogeneous cancer. Premalignancies display fluctuating levels of dissimilar hereditary, sub-atomic, and transcriptomic profiles contrasted with both ordinary tissue and threatening cancers, notwithstanding, a few pieces of information recommend that this is reliant upon obtrusive potential. Explicit models from the bosom and esophageal cancer complement the need of

figuring out this changeability. Studies using bosom cell lines have shown unmistakable articulation marks happening along the range of ordinary to obtrusive carcinomas; a significant number of the distinguished changes were epigenetic. Moreover, the transcriptomic profiles of ladies were significantly unique between the individuals who created bosom disease as long as 5 years before determination and ladies who were cancer-free, recommending that a considerable lot of these modifications happen preceding cancer commencement and preparing of the threatening specialty. Comparative examples of hereditary modifications have been seen in Barrett's throat, a known forerunner sore to esophageal adenocarcinoma, and colorectal adenomas, which can change into adenocarcinomas. Non-dysplastic Barrett's throat has a lower mutational weight (5.4-6.8 single nucleotide varieties per megabase) contrasted with dysplastic Barrett's throat, which, thusly, has a lower mutational weight than esophageal adenocarcinoma. Furthermore, a few transformations have been planned across the ordinary to threatening range. Repetitive transformations in TP53 have been seen in high-grade dysplastic Barrett's throat and esophageal adenocarcinoma, but SMAD4 changes have just been seen in obtrusive lesions. The differential profiles of cancer through tumorigenesis beginning at early sores to cutting edge/intrusive sickness might give a one-of-a-kind road to early identification, especially on the off chance that we can pinpoint explicitly which early occasions prompt disease movement. Be that as it may, sub-atomic profiling of early injuries can be a costly undertaking as an unmistakable greater part of premalignant sore don't advance to intrusive cancer, and an inexorably bigger example size is expected to distinguish drivers of movement as we push toward early precancerous injuries.
Early cancer identification modalities, like mammography, colonoscopy, prostate-explicit antigen (PSA) screening, and cervical cell cytology (Pap smear), have been generally carried out. Mammography is an acknowledged practice with moderately high adherence in regions where assets are accessible. However mammography is viewed as the 'highest quality level' for bosom cancer early identification at a reparable stage, but it isn't without its expenses. Misleading up-sides, which prompts superfluous patient biopsies, and overdiagnosis, which is the identification of injuries that would eventually not prompt cancer-related passing, happen at a high rate. Essentially, routine PSA testing for the identification of prostate cancer in the United States has brought about a comparative result, causing superfluous development and overtreatment. Extraordinary Britain, which doesn't constantly involve PSA for screening, has practically identical prostate cancer rates to the United States, scrutinizing the utility of PSA for the early identification of prostate disease.
Notwithstanding issues, there have been a few victories in cancer screening. A significant achievement was the execution and scattering of cervical cancer cytology screening, or Pap spreads. This negligibly obtrusive screening methodology considers the immediate representation of cell changes happening in the cervix, which can then be utilized to fittingly illuminate treatment choices, for example, colposcopy or cryotherapy. The aftereffects of Pap spreads alone, be that as it may, can be inconvenient. A demonstrating concentrate on researching cervical cancer results in the Dutch library assessed that roughly 74% of cervical diseases were a consequence of overdiagnosis. When matched with HPV testing, the general results get to the next level. In this manner, while carrying out and assessing cancer counteraction procedures, it is important to consider and streamline the gamble benefit proportion of the philosophy and breaking point the chance of unjustifiable mischief to the patient populace.

The case for the accuracy of Cancer prevention

A significant collection of exploration has been committed to researching the pathways associated with cancer commencement, movement, and metastasis, and distinguishing biomarkers related to these instruments for clinical utility. The term 'biomarker', be that as it may, is expansive and incorporates a large number of natural highlights or particles, like imaging or radio mic modifications, DNA adjustments, articulation of various RNA types, and metabolomic and proteomic changes. No matter what the biomarker type, the ideal biomarker ought to be: (1) straightforwardly connected with the sickness of interest, (2) be associated with something like one piece of the cancer range, (3) give high responsiveness and particularity, (4) have moderately harmless identification, and 5) have a sensible money saving advantage proportion. The outcome of individual biomarkers has been restricted, but progress has been utilized biomarker boards for the early identification and accuracy therapy of a few cancer, like bosom disease and melanoma. The American Society for Clinical Oncology suggests cancer composing of estrogen receptor (ER), progesterone receptor (PR), and human epidermal development factor receptor 2 (HER2) in bosom biopsies. The data accomplished from this growth composing can then be utilized to illuminate interventive choices, like tamoxifen for ER-positive diseases, trastuzumab for HER2-positive tumors, or the requirement for extra hereditary investigation. A comparative layered approach can be used in the early identification of melanoma holding onto BRAF-V600E transformations. Roughly half of the melanomas have a transformation in BRAF which brings about the constitutive enactment of the Ras/Raf/MEK pathway. Of these, more than 90% of the BRAF transformations are a missense change bringing about the replacement of valine for glutamic corrosive at codon 600. Early identification of melanoma and growth composing for the BRAF-V600E transformation can then illuminate restorative choices, for example, treatment with vemurafenib or dabrafenib which explicitly focus on the initiating change.

In a perfect world, be that as it may, biomarkers ought to be utilized to decide the possible viability of a cancer counteraction methodology, as opposed to holding on until show and determination. One such model is the utilization of anti-inflammatory medicine for the counteraction of colorectal cancer. However the utilization of low-portion day-to-day anti-inflammatory medicine is for the most part suggested for more established people (age 50-69) with explicit cardiovascular sickness risk, ibuprofen use has exhibited expanded viability for colorectal cancer counteraction in comparative age bunch people with unmistakable biomarkers. For instance, a settled case-control examination of the Nurses' Health Study and the Health Professional Follow-up Study, two enormous imminent companion studies, discovered that people with the single nucleotide polymorphism (SNP) rs6983267 T allele in CTNNB1, which codes for the protein β-catenin, impacts the development of the Wnt/β-catenin obliteration complex. Anti-inflammatory medicine diminished β-catenin articulation, which thusly restrains record and initiation of MYC, decreasing colorectal cancer potential. Then again, at a similar area in CTNNB1 the replacement to a G allele, as opposed to a T allele, brings about an expanded obliteration complex restricting and may advance colorectal disease movement. A comparative relationship of diminished colorectal cancer risk has been noticed for the SNPs rs2965667 (TT) in MGST1 and rs16973225 (AA) situated close to IL16.

Tragically, the reconciliation of such sub-atomic components for the early identification and therapy of cancer isn't far-reaching, however genomic characterization of different diseases might prompt enhancements in cancer counteraction methodologies and assist with distinguishing high-risk people. Especially, the genomic portrayal of cancer might pinpoint significant modifications which can then be utilized for designated intercessions. Evaluating suggestions for colorectal cancer have rotated around a comparative methodology. Ebb and flow evaluating rules for colorectal cancer delineate people into four gamble gatherings: (1) a high-risk bunch, which incorporates inherited conditions, for example, familial adenomatous polyposis and Lynch disorder, (2) a moderate-risk bunch, which incorporates obtained expanded risk conditions, like provocative entrail infection or colitis, (3) a typical gamble bunch (for example people beyond 45 50 and 4 years old), a generally safe gathering that prohibits the other illustrated gatherings. Notwithstanding delineation, there remains intergroup heterogeneity, alluding to various degrees of individual infection risk inside a separated gathering, which might be moved toward by additional definition of chance variables inside each gathering. Examination of a gambling record for the improvement of cutting edge neoplasia in normal gambling people utilizing the way of life and conduct factors, for example, weight file (BMI) and smoking status, can distinguish low-and high-risk people inside this gathering. This data might be additionally used to exhort screening methodologies.

Considering this methodology, the Women Informed to Screen Depending on Measures of Risk (WISDOM) study was intended to sober-mindedly research yearly versus risk-based evaluation for bosom cancer. Just 10% of ladies have a precise impression of their gamble for bosom cancer and 40% of ladies have never talked about their gamble of bosom disease with their primary care physician. The WISDOM preliminary looks to lay out the viability of hazard-based screening, which incorporates clinical gamble factors (for example BMI, age), bosom thickness, and polygenic gamble score, contrasted with yearly evaluation for bosom cancer, which is not entirely set in stone through the number of biopsies performed and estimation of member horribleness. However the consummation and investigation of the WISDOM preliminary is a long way from getting done, this study might move the needle to start incorporating accurate risk-based evaluating methodologies for specific cancer.

Quick logical and innovative advances ought to take into consideration a more precise delineation of in-danger people who might profit from counteraction methodologies. This might incorporate expanded screening or reconnaissance, elective medicines, or early forceful treatment. This technique may likewise include diminished evaluating or reconnaissance for generally safe gatherings. A functioning gathering researching the utility of accuracy risk delineation based evaluation and proposals for colorectal cancer from the United States Military Health System recommended barring generally safe people from screening that might probably be relieved by careful intercession alone, distinguish and locally treat patients with beginning phase CRC, and limit medicines to patients with inactive or stable infection.

Accuracy prevention

As the optimistic objective of cancer counteraction is to restrain the development of disease preceding commencement, essential anticipation is basic to achieve this objective. Accuracy counteraction consolidates accuracy medication draws near and the people's gamble profile, which is characterized by genomic and way of life risk factors. The ongoing period of logical development has distinguished a few strategies that might be serendipitous, fundamentally in the early identification of cancer and take advantage of hereditary gamble factors. For example, circling without cell DNA (cfDNA) can be disconnected from plasma, serum, pee, or other body liquids as a substitute biomarker (for example mSEPT9, KRAS, and CDKN2A), to look at generally speaking infection trouble, or perform Next-age sequencing to foster hereditary profiles. For the most part, raised degrees of cfDNA and coursing growth DNA (ctDNA) can be distinguished foundationally in patients with the disease, but cfDNA isn't well defined for cancer and might be connected with different pathologies. Then again, as cfDNA can be sequenced, the disclosure of hereditary distortions, like transformations (e.g., in KRAS, TP53, or APC or frameshifts in microsatellites) may give a more exact device to distinguish the presence of right on time or beforehand undetected cancer. Additionally, ctDNA and coursing growth cells (CTCs) can be disconnected from plasma or serum and evaluated for sub-atomic modifications. For instance, Morelli and associates inspected pre-and post-therapy plasma from patients with metastatic colorectal cancer and showed distinguishable EGFR and KRAS transformations. Identification of EGFR after treatment corresponded with lower movement-free endurance. Be that as it may, the identification of ctDNA and CTCs is at present not dependable for recognition of either beginning phase sickness because of a scarcity of cancer cells in precancers; in any case, this procedure has exhibited some utility in anticipating the hazard of repeat after therapy. The ease of use of cfDNA, ctDNA, and CTCs for the early identification of cancer has been guaranteed, yet there are a few restrictions to these procedures. The portrayed techniques have little viability in distinguishing premalignant or beginning phase sickness because of the low foundational overflow of the marker and restrictions in examining responsiveness and reproducibility. Different issues, like fluctuating articulation between people, may influence the unwavering quality of cancer biomarkers. The biomarker of interest may not be well defined for growth cells and delivered by typical or non-carcinogenic cells, may not be created by early injuries, or may not be delivered by all cancer cells. Along these lines, there are a few situations wherein early injuries might miss by the screen. Moreover, similarly, as with every single new innovation, execution of these identification modalities is at present not plausible for an enormous scope. Most clinical focuses don't have the assets accessible to play out the measures fundamental for the assessment of cfDNA, ctDNA, or CTCs. In addition to the fact that these examines be tentatively difficult and display high can changeability, for the precise early identification of cancer we should likewise know the fundamental sub-atomic abnormalities of the sickness for recognition. However, there are high recurrence hereditary changes that happen ahead of schedule in carcinogenesis for specific cancer, and the genomic scene of disease is tremendous. The extraordinary hereditary qualities of a people's growth convolute our capacity to foster modalities to distinguish profiles appropriately. With the continuous improvement of the Human Tumor Atlas and the Precancer Atlas, the information on these infection states and potential hereditary targets is extending, however, is at present beyond populace level achievability.

The eventual fate of accuracy screening and prevention

We should initially inquire: is cancer counteraction fundamentally exact? The following intelligent inquiry is: does it matter? A few suggested cancer counteraction methodologies have exhibited significant viability pussyfoot around the possibility of accuracy. Long haul utilization of non-steroidal mitigating drugs (NSAIDs) and cyclooxygenase-2 inhibitors (COXIBs) have been related to a diminished gamble of fostering a few gastrointestinal cancers, however, an inhibitory impact has been noticed reliably in colorectal disease. NSAID and COXIB use has been compelling in diminishing the occurrence of adenomas and colorectal cancer in both genetic/high-chance and normal gamble populaces. The United States Preventative Services Task Force (USPSTF) has incorporated an accurate counteraction approach into the populace-level proof-based suggestions. For people ages 50-59 with a long haul (>10 years) endanger of cardiovascular infection and a future of something like 10 years who will take low-portion headache medicine day to day and are not in danger of dying, the USPSTF suggests the utilization of low-portion ibuprofen for the counteraction of both cardiovascular sickness and colorectal cancer. This suggestion changes for people between the ages of 60-69, to such an extent that the choice ought to be private. Additionally, for those over 69 years of age, there is no suggestion to involve anti-inflammatory medicine as the information is at present lacking. The general rules (for example long haul hazard of cardiovascular infection, not at expanded chance of dying) continue as before, but the choice to start day-to-day low-portion headache medicine ought to happen on a singular premise.

NSAIDs and COXIBs have shown sensible viability as cancer counteraction specialists for gastrointestinal diseases, however, can this be viewed as accuracy anticipation? NSAIDs restrain cyclooxygenase (COX)−1 and COX-2, diminishing prostaglandin biosynthesis and aggravation. COXIBs act through a comparative instrument and explicitly target COX-2. Along these lines, utilization of NSAIDs and COXIBs don't simply decrease gastrointestinal aggravation, but foundational irritation. Maybe the commencement and movement of gastrointestinal cancer are more reliant upon persevering aggravation contrasted with other essential cancer destinations. This can be construed from the relationship between persistent provocative infections, like incendiary entrail sickness and Crohn's illness, and expanded risk for colorectal cancer. Corpulence is likewise connected with persistent irritation, which might assume a part in the viability of headache medicine in forestalling colorectal cancer. Rothwell and partners as of late researched the impact of headache medicine on the gamble of cardiovascular occasions and cancer in an aggregate of randomized preliminaries and found that the protection impact of ibuprofen on disease risk is reliant upon bodyweight and portion. On the off chance that this can be affirmed in resulting studies, this perception requires a customized portion or potentially routine of headache medicine and most likely other cancer preventives in light of body weight. Comparative affiliations have been seen between Helicobactor pylori contamination and gastric cancer, esophagitis and esophageal adenocarcinoma, and pancreatitis and pancreatic disease. NSAIDs and COXIBs' capability to unequivocally smother aggravation, yet the effect is foundational and not conclusively expected for the particular gamble decrease of gastrointestinal cancer.

The relationship between NSAID or COXIB use and the diminished chance of gastrointestinal cancer, however not other disease types, features a significant detail that fundamentally influences accuracy counteraction: cancer heterogeneity. For this situation, cancer heterogeneity not just alludes to varieties in hereditary and sub-atomic profiles between and inside growth types, yet additionally the conduct and ecological variables and the natural modifications that guide the commencement and movement of malignancies. Some cancer counteraction specialists can be all the more stringently delegated an accuracy counteraction specialist. Tamoxifen and raloxifene are particular estrogen receptor modulators (SERMs) and have exhibited critical viability in the counteraction of ER-positive bosom cancer. In any case, in light of the fact that these specialists, as well as aromatase inhibitors, target chemical receptors which are organ-explicit, their viability is restricted to cancers that express ER and are not especially advantageous against the other bosom disease subtypes. The Breast Cancer Prevention Trial P-1, Multiple Outcomes of Raloxifene Evaluation, and Study of Tamoxifen and Raloxifene (STAR) preliminaries researched the viability of SERMs to forestall the improvement of bosom cancer in dangerous ladies (for example post-menopausal, more than 35 years of age). These preliminaries exhibited a decrease of intrusive bosom cancer occurrence by 49%, 70%, and 44-90%, individually. Be that as it may, the STAR preliminary showed an expanded gamble of uterine

cancer among people given tamoxifen, in this manner demonstrating expected mischief of SERMs for counteraction. To possibly neutralize the inconvenient impact of foundational SERMs, an ongoing bosom cancer counteraction preliminary is researching the viability of effective utilization of tamoxifen, taking into consideration restricted counteraction.
A comparative contention can be made for other disease counteraction specialists with specific sub-atomic targets, for example, the epidermal development factor receptor (EGFR) inhibitor erlotinib for the counteraction of head and neck cancer. Erlotinib, in blend with celecoxib, was utilized in a Phase Ib/pharmacokinetic investigation of head and neck cancer counteraction among people with oral leukoplakia, dysplasia, and carcinoma in situ. However, the preliminary exhibited introductory viability and the greater part of the premalignant injuries were repeated or advanced. The Erlotinib Prevention of Oral Cancer (EPOC) preliminary, a randomized, fake treatment controlled, twofold visually impaired preliminary which utilized loss of heterozygosity and EGFR duplicate number to delineate and assess patients, likewise missing the mark on clinical proof to help the utilization of erlotinib for head and neck cancer counteraction, as EGFR articulation couldn't anticipate erlotinib viability. Except if the overexpression, initiation, or transformation of the sub-atomic objective is reliably constitutively communicated across and inside cancer types and is fundamental for carcinogenesis, all-inclusive disease counteraction with a solitary specialist is a troublesome obstacle to survival. Regardless of whether the marker is constitutively communicated, there is no assurance that the designated specialist will demonstrate effectiveness. Besides, with the expansion of additional specialists expected to accomplish precaution esteem through synergistic activity, the gamble of unsatisfactory poison levels increments, especially for specialists requiring long haul dosing.
In cancer counteraction, does accuracy matter? At times, at the point when we can tie explicit hereditary variables, for example, epigenetic or hereditary modifications, and other non-hereditary elements, like family ancestry, to precisely evaluate one's gamble of a specific sort or subset of cancer, accuracy screening, reconnaissance, and counteraction is a valuable methodology as we can change risk-benefit profiles in light of the gamble of obtrusive disease. On the other hand, for a significant part of the populace who are people at normal gamble for cancer improvement, using the more worldwide disease protection measures, for example, NSAIDs, changing way of life factors (for example diet, exercise, and tobacco use), and screening, may eventually demonstrate more advantageous. In this manner, we really want to all the more likely distinguish a delineation methodology where the gamble benefit proportion is positive in people with an expanded gamble of cancer or who have an expanded gamble of openings to disease-causing substances, and that people with generally safe bring about negligible mischief. However summed enemy of cancer drives is not exact, these strategies can arrive at a bigger populace and extend their effect. Evaluating and distinguishing the effect of various cancer types will give data on focusing on disease counteraction drives and methodologies, whether those techniques are based at the individual-or populace level.

Immunotherapy to Treat Cancer

Immunotherapy is a sort of cancer therapy that assists your insusceptible framework with battling disease. The insusceptible framework assists your body with battling contaminations and different sicknesses. It is comprised of white platelets and organs and tissues of the lymph framework.
Immunotherapy is a kind of organic treatment. Natural treatment is a kind of therapy that utilizes substances produced using living organic entities to treat cancer.

ON THIS PAGE WE'LL BE LOOKING AT

- How does immunotherapy neutralize cancer?
- What are the kinds of immunotherapy?
- Which cancers are treated with immunotherapy?
- What are the symptoms of immunotherapy?
- How is immunotherapy given?
- Where do you go for immunotherapy?
- How frequently do you get immunotherapy?
- How might you let me know if immunotherapy is working?
- What is the ebb and flow of research in immunotherapy?

How immunotherapy neutralizes Cancer?

As a component of its generally expected capability, the insusceptible framework distinguishes and obliterates unusual cells and in all probability forestalls or controls the development of numerous cancers. For example, resistant cells are some of the time viewed in and around cancers. These phones, called cancer penetrating lymphocytes or TILs, are an indication that the insusceptible framework is answering the growth. Individuals whose cancers contain TILs frequently show improvement over individuals whose growths don't contain them.

Despite the fact that the insusceptible framework can forestall or slow disease development, cancer cells have ways of keeping away from annihilation by the invulnerable framework. For instance, cancer cells may:

• Have hereditary changes that make them less noticeable to the insusceptible framework.

• Have proteins on their surface that mood killer insusceptible cells.

• Change the ordinary cells around the growth so they slow down how the insusceptible framework answers the disease cells.

Immunotherapy assists the insusceptible framework with bettering demonstration against cancer.

Kinds of immunotherapies

A few kinds of immunotherapy are utilized to treat cancer. These include:

• Insusceptible designated spot inhibitors, which are drugs that block invulnerable designated spots. These designated spots are an ordinary piece of the insusceptible framework and hold invulnerable reactions back from being serious areas of strength excessively. By obstructing them, these medications permit insusceptible cells to answer all the more unequivocally to cancer.

How do insusceptible designated spot inhibitors neutralize cancer?

Insusceptible designated spots are an ordinary piece of the invulnerable framework. Their job is to keep a resistant reaction from being solid to such an extent that it obliterates sound cells in the body.

Insusceptible designated spots connect with when proteins on the outer layer of invulnerable cells called T cells perceive and tie to accomplice proteins on different cells, like some growth cells. These proteins are called insusceptible designated spot proteins. At the point when the designated spot and accomplice proteins tie together, they send an "off" motion toward the T cells. This can keep the insusceptible framework from annihilating cancer.

Immunotherapy drugs called insusceptible designated spot inhibitors work by obstructing designated spot proteins from restricting their accomplice proteins. This forestalls the "off" signal from being sent, permitting the T cells to kill cancer cells.
One such medication acts against a designated spot protein called CTLA-4. Other insusceptible designated spot inhibitors act against a designated spot protein called PD-1 or its accomplice protein PD-L1. A few cancers turn down the T cell reaction by delivering bunches of PD-L1.

Cancers that are treated with insusceptible designated spot inhibitors

Insusceptible designated spot inhibitors are supported to treat certain individuals with an assortment of Cancer types, including:

- Bosom cancer
- Bladder cancer
- Cervical cancer
- Colon cancer
- Head and neck cancer
- Hodgkin lymphoma
- Liver cancer
- Cellular breakdown in the lungs
- Renal cell cancer (a sort of kidney disease)
- Skin cancer, including melanoma
- Rectal cancer
- Any strong cancer that can't fix blunders in DNA happen when the DNA is duplicated

What incidental effects are brought about by insusceptible designated spot inhibitors?

Resistant designated spot inhibitors can cause secondary effects that influence individuals in various ways. The incidental effect you might have and how they affect you will rely heavily on how sound you are before therapy, your kind of cancer, how cutting-edge it is, the sort of insusceptible designated spot inhibitor you are getting, and the portion.
Specialists and medical caretakers can't be aware without a doubt when or on the other hand on the off chance that incidental effects will happen or how serious they will be. Along these lines, it is essential to realize which signs to search for and what to do on the off chance that they happen.

Normal symptoms of insusceptible designated spot inhibitors include:

- Rash
- Looseness of the bowels
- Exhaustion

More extraordinary symptoms of insusceptible designated spot inhibitors can incorporate far and wide aggravation. Contingent upon the organ of your body that is impacted, aggravation can prompt:

- Changes in skin tone, rash, and feeling bothersome, brought about by skin aggravation
- Hack and chest torments, brought about by aggravation in the lungs
- Midsection torment and looseness of the bowels, brought about by aggravation in the colon
- Diabetes, brought about by aggravation in the pancreas
- Hepatitis (aggravation of the liver)
- Hypophysitis (aggravation of the pituitary organ)

• Myocarditis (aggravation of the heart muscle)
• Nephritis (aggravation of the kidney) and debilitated kidney capability
• Overactive or underactive thyroid
• Sensory system issues like muscle shortcoming, deadness, and inconvenience relaxing
• Immune system microorganism move treatment, which is a therapy that supports the inherent capacity of your T cells to battle cancer. In this treatment, resistant cells are taken from your growth. Those that are generally dynamic against your cancer are chosen or changed in the lab to all the more likely to assault your disease cells, filled in enormous clusters, and set back into your body through a needle in a vein.

Lymphocyte move treatment may likewise be called supportive cell treatment, assenting immunotherapy, or insusceptible cell treatment.

How does T-cell move treatment neutralize cancer?

Lymphocyte move treatment is a sort of immunotherapy that improves your own insusceptible cells ready to go after cancer. There are two fundamental sorts of T-cell move treatment: cancer penetrating lymphocytes (or TIL) treatment and CAR T-cell treatment. Both include gathering your own resistant cells, developing enormous quantities of these phones in the lab, and afterward giving the phones back to you through a needle in your vein. Lymphocyte move treatment is additionally called supportive cell treatment, assenting immunotherapy, and insusceptible cell treatment.

The most common way of developing your T cells in the lab can require 2 to about two months. During this time, you might have therapy with chemotherapy and, perhaps, radiation treatment to dispose of other insusceptible cells. Diminishing your insusceptible cells helps the moved T cells to be more compelling. After these medicines, the T cells that were filled in the lab will be rewarded to you by means of a needle in your vein.

• Until treatment utilizes T cells called growth penetrating lymphocytes that are tracked down in your cancer. Specialists test these lymphocytes in the lab to figure out which ones best perceive your cancer cells. Then, at that point, these chosen lymphocytes are treated with substances that cause them to develop in enormous numbers rapidly.

The thought behind this approach is that the lymphocytes that are in or close to the growth have proactively shown the capacity to perceive your cancer cells. In any case, there may not be enough of them to kill cancer or to conquer the signs that the growth is delivering to smother the resistant framework. Giving you enormous quantities of the lymphocytes that respond best with the growth can assist with conquering these obstructions.

• CAR T-cell treatment is like TIL treatment, however, your T cells are changed in the lab so they spread the word about a kind of protein like CAR before they are developed and rewarded you. CARs represent Chimeric Antigen Receptor. CARs are intended to permit the T cells to connect to explicit proteins on the outer layer of the cancer cells, working on their capacity to go after the disease cells.

What cancers are treated with T-cell move treatment?

White blood cell move treatment was first read up for the treatment of metastatic melanoma since melanomas frequently cause serious areas of strength for a reaction and frequently have numerous TILs. The utilization of TIL treatment has been compelling for certain individuals with melanoma and has delivered promising discoveries in different cancer, for example, cervical squamous cell carcinoma and cholangiocarcinoma. Be that as it may, this treatment is as yet exploratory.

Six CAR T-cell treatments have been supported by the Food and Drug Administration for blood cancer.

- Axicabtagene Ciloleucel (Yescarta™)
- Brexucabtagene autoleucel (Tecartus™)
- Ciltacabtagene autoleucel (Carvykti™)
- Iidecabtagene vicleucel (Abecma™)
- Ilisocabtagene maraleucel (Breyanzi™)
- Tisagenlecleucel (Kymriah™)

Car T-cell treatment has additionally been read up for the therapy of strong growths, including bosom and cerebrum diseases, however, use in such cancer is as yet exploratory.

Symptoms of T-cell move treatment

Immune system microorganism move treatment can cause secondary effects, which individuals experience in various ways. The incidental effects you might have and how serious they are will rely heavily on how solid you are before therapy, your kind of cancer, how cutting-edge it is, the sort of T-cell move treatment you are getting, and the portion.

Specialists and medical attendants can't be aware without a doubt when or on the other hand on the off chance that incidental effects will happen or what they will mean for you. Along these lines, it is essential to realize which signs to search for and what to do on the off chance that you begin to have issues.

Car T-cell treatment can cause a serious incidental effect known as cytokine discharge condition. This condition is caused when the moved T cells, or other insusceptible cells answering the new T cells, discharge a lot of cytokines into the blood.

Cytokines are resistant substances that have a wide range of capabilities in the body. An unexpected expansion in their levels can cause:

- Fever
- Nausea
- Cerebral pain
- Rash
- Quick heartbeat
- Low circulatory strain
- Inconvenience relaxing

A great many people have a gentle type of cytokine discharge condition. Be that as it may, in certain individuals, it very well might be serious or hazardous.

Additionally, in spite of the fact that CAR T cells are intended to perceive proteins that are found exclusively on cancer cells, they can likewise some of the time perceive ordinary cells.

Contingent upon which ordinary cells are perceived, this can cause a scope of incidental effects, including organ harm.

Until treatment can cause hair-like break condition, this condition makes liquid and proteins spill out of minuscule veins and stream into encompassing tissues, bringing about hazardously low circulatory strain. Hair-like break conditions might prompt different organ disappointment and shock.

Monoclonal antibodies

Are resistant framework proteins made in labs that are intended to tie to an explicit focus on cancer cells. A few monoclonal antibodies mark cancer cells with the goal that they will be better seen and obliterated by the insusceptible framework. Such monoclonal antibodies are a sort of immunotherapy.

Monoclonal antibodies may likewise be called restorative antibodies.

How do monoclonal antibodies neutralize cancer?

Monoclonal antibodies are resistant framework proteins that are made in the lab. Antibodies are delivered normally by your body and assist the insusceptible framework with perceiving microorganisms that cause infection, like microscopic organisms and infections, and imprint them for obliteration. Like your body's own antibodies, monoclonal antibodies perceive explicit targets.

Numerous monoclonal antibodies are utilized to treat cancer. They are a kind of designated cancer treatment, and that implies they are intended to collaborate with explicit targets.

A few monoclonal antibodies are likewise immunotherapy since they assist with turning the insusceptible framework against cancer. For instance, a few monoclonal antibodies mark cancer cells with the goal that the insusceptible framework will better perceive and obliterate them. A model is a rituximab, which ties to a protein called CD20 on B cells and a few sorts of cancer cells, making the insusceptible framework kill them. B cells are a sort of white platelet.

Other monoclonal antibodies bring T cells near cancer cells, assisting the insusceptible cells with killing the disease cells. A model is a blinatumomab (Blincyto®), which ties to both CD19, a protein tracked down on the outer layer of leukemia cells, and CD3, a protein on the outer layer of T cells. This interaction assists the T cells with drawing near enough to the leukemia cells to answer and kill them.

A few monoclonal antibodies bring immune system microorganisms near cancer cells, assisting them with killing disease cells.

Which cancer is treated with monoclonal antibodies?

Numerous monoclonal antibodies have been supported to treat a wide assortment of cancer.

Symptoms of monoclonal antibodies

Monoclonal antibodies can cause incidental effects, which can contrast from one individual to another. The ones you might have and how they affect you will rely upon many variables, for example, how solid you are before therapy, your kind of cancer, how cutting-edge it is, the sort of monoclonal counteracting agent you are getting, and the portion.

Specialists and medical attendants can't be aware without a doubt when or on the other hand on the off chance that incidental effects will happen or how serious they will be. Along these lines, it is essential to realize which signs to search for and what to do on the off chance that you begin to have issues.

Like most sorts of immunotherapy, monoclonal antibodies can cause skin responses at the needle site and influenza-like side effects.

Needle site responses include:

- Torment
- Expanding

• Irritation
• Redness
• Irritation
• Rash

Influenza-like side effects include:
• Chills
• Exhaustion
• Fever
• Muscle a throbbing painfulness
• Nausea
• Regurgitating
• Looseness of the bowels

Monoclonal antibodies can likewise cause:
• Mouth and skin injuries that can prompt serious contaminations
• Hypertension
• Congestive cardiovascular breakdown
• Cardiovascular failures
• Provocative lung infection

Monoclonal antibodies can cause gentle to serious unfavorably susceptible responses while you are getting the medication. In uncommon cases, the response is sufficiently extreme to cause passing.

A few monoclonal antibodies can likewise cause hair like break conditions. This condition makes liquid and proteins spill out of minuscule veins and stream into encompassing tissues, bringing about hazardously low circulatory strain. Hair like break conditions might prompt different organ disappointment and shock.

Cytokine discharge condition can some of the time happen with monoclonal antibodies; however, it is frequently gentle. Cytokines are resistant substances that have a wide range of capabilities in the body, and an unexpected expansion in their levels can cause:
• Fever
• Nausea
• Cerebral pain
• Rash
• Quick heartbeat
• Low circulatory strain
• Inconvenience relaxing
• Therapy immunizations, which neutralize cancer by supporting your insusceptible framework's reaction to disease cells. Treatment immunizations are unique in relation to the ones that assist with forestalling sickness.

How do Cancer therapy immunizations neutralize disease?

Cancer therapy immunizations are a sort of immunotherapy that treats disease by reinforcing the body's regular protection against cancer. Not all cancer counteraction immunizations, disease therapy antibodies are intended to be utilized in individuals who as of now have cancer they neutralize cancer cells, not against something that causes cancer.

The thought behind therapy immunizations is that cancer contains substances, called cancer-related antigens, that are absent in typical cells or on the other hand, assuming present, are at lower levels. Therapy immunizations can assist the insusceptible framework with figuring out how to perceive and respond to these antigens and obliterate cancer cells that contain them.

Fundamental ways Cancer treatment immunizations might be made in.
1. They can be produced using your own growth cells. This implies they are specially designed so they cause an insusceptible reaction against highlights that are one of a kind to your cancer.
2. They might be produced using growth-related antigens that are tracked down on disease cells of many individuals with a particular sort of cancer. Such an immunization can cause a resistant reaction in any understanding whose cancer delivers that antigen. This kind of immunization is as yet exploratory.
3. They might be produced using your own dendritic cells, which are a kind of insusceptible cells. Dendritic cell immunizations invigorate your insusceptible framework to answer an antigen on growth cells. One dendritic cell immunization has been supported, sipuleucel-T, which is utilized to treat a few men with cutting-edge prostate cancer.

An alternate kind of cancer therapy, called oncolytic infection treatment, is some of the time portrayed as a sort of disease treatment immunization. It utilizes an oncolytic infection, which is an infection that contaminates and separates cancer cells but doesn't hurt ordinary cells.

The principal FDA-supported oncolytic infection treatment is talimogene laherparepvec (T-VEC, or Imlygic®). It depends on herpes simplex infection type 1. Albeit this infection can contaminate both cancer and ordinary cells, typical cells can kill the infection while disease cells can't.

T-VEC is infused straightforwardly into cancer. As the infection makes an ever-increasing number of duplicates of itself, it makes cancer cells burst and kick the bucket. The withering cells discharge new infections and different substances that can cause an insusceptible reaction against cancer cells all through the body.

Which cancer is treated with cancer treatment immunizations?
Sipuleucel-T is utilized to treat individuals with prostate cancer:
• That has spread to different pieces of the body
• Who have little or no side effects
• Whose cancer doesn't answer chemical treatment

T-VEC is utilized to treat certain individuals with melanoma that profits after surgery and can't be eliminated with more surgery.

Symptoms of Cancer treatment immunizations
Cancer treatment immunizations can cause secondary effects, which influence individuals in various ways. The incidental effect you may have and how they affect you will rely heavily on how sound you are before therapy, your sort of cancer, how cutting-edge it is, the kind of treatment immunization you are getting, and the portion.

Specialists and medical attendants can't be aware without a doubt when or on the other hand on the off chance that incidental effects will happen or how serious they will be. Along these lines, it is essential to realize which signs to search for and what to do on the off chance that you begin to have issues.

Cancer treatment immunizations can cause influenza-like side effects, which include:

- Fever
- Chills
- Shortcoming
- Nausea or regurgitating
- Muscle or joint throbs
- Exhaustion
- Cerebral pain
- Inconvenience relaxing
- Low or hypertension

Get more familiar with influenza-like side effects brought about by cancer treatment.

You might have an extreme unfavorably susceptible response.

Sipuleucel-T can cause a stroke.

T-VEC can cause growth lysis conditions. In this condition, the growth cells kick the bucket and fall to pieces in the blood. This changes specific synthetic substances in the blood, which might make harm organs like the kidneys, heart, and liver.

Since T-VEC is produced using herpesvirus it can some of the time cause herpes virus contamination that can prompt:

- Torment, consuming, or shivering in a rankle around the mouth, private parts, fingers, or ears
- Eye torment, responsiveness, release from the eyes, and foggy vision
- Shortcoming in the arms and legs
- Outrageous exhaustion and sluggishness
- Disarray
- Insusceptible framework modulators, which improve the body's invulnerable reaction against cancer. A portion of these specialists influences explicit pieces of the resistant framework, though others influence the safe framework in a broader manner.

How do insusceptible framework modulators neutralize cancer?

Insusceptible regulating specialists are a kind of immunotherapy that improves the body's invulnerable reaction against cancer.

Sorts of insusceptible regulating specialists include:

- Cytokines are proteins made by white platelets. They assume significant parts in your body's ordinary resistant reactions and in the safe framework's capacity to answer cancer.

Cytokines that are some of the time used to treat cancer include:

- **Interferons** (INFs). Specialists have tracked down that one sort of interferon, called INF-alfa, can upgrade your insusceptible reaction to cancer cells by prompting specific white platelets, like regular executioner cells and dendritic cells, to become dynamic. INF-alfa may likewise sluggish the development of cancer cells or advance their passing.

- **Interleukins** (ILs). There are in excess of twelve interleukins, including IL-2, which is additionally called the T-cell development factor. IL-2 lifts the number of white platelets in the body, including executioner T cells and regular executioner cells. Expanding these cells can

cause an insusceptible reaction against cancer. IL-2 additionally helps B cells (one more kind of white platelet) produce specific substances that can target cancer cells.
Hematopoietic development factors are cytokines that are utilized to decrease incidental effects from disease treatment by advancing the development of platelets that are harmed by chemotherapy. They include:
Erythropoietin, which expands the development of red platelets
- IL-11, which expands the development of platelets
- **Granulocyte-macrophage settlement invigorating component (GM-CSF) and granulocyte province animating variable (G-CSF),** which both increment the number of white platelets. Supporting white platelets diminishes the gamble of contaminations. G-CSF and GM-CSF can likewise upgrade the insusceptible framework reaction against disease by expanding the quantity of cancer-battling T cells.
- **BCG** is a debilitating type of microscopic organism that causes tuberculosis. It doesn't cause sickness in people. BCG is utilized to treat bladder cancer. When embedded straightforwardly into the bladder with a catheter, BCG causes an insusceptible reaction against cancer cells. It is additionally being concentrated on in different sorts of cancer. BCG represents Bacillus Calmette-Guérin.
  Immunomodulatory drugs (additionally called organic reaction modifiers) invigorate the insusceptible frameworks which include:
- Thalidomide (Thalomid®)
- Lenalidomide (Revlimid®)
- Pomalidomide (Pomalyst®)
- Imiquimod (Aldara®, Zyclara®)

Thalidomide, lenaliodomide, and pomalidomide make cells discharge IL-2. They additionally prevent cancers from shaping fresh blood vessels. Cancers need to frame fresh blood vessels to develop past a specific size. These three medications may likewise be called angiogenesis inhibitors.
Imiquimod is a cream that you rub on the skin. It makes cells discharge cytokines.

Cancer is treated with insusceptible framework modulators
Most insusceptible regulating specialists are utilized to treat progressed cancer. Some are utilized to assist with overseeing incidental effects.
What are the symptoms of insusceptible framework modulators?
Resistant regulating specialists can cause secondary effects, which influence individuals in various ways. The incidental effect you might have and how they affect you will rely heavily on how sound you are before therapy, your sort of cancer, how cutting-edge it is, the kind of insusceptible regulating specialist you are getting, and the portion.
Specialists and medical attendants can't be aware without a doubt when or on the other hand on the off chance that incidental effects will happen or how serious they will be. Along these lines, it is essential to realize which signs to search for and what to do on the off chance that you begin to have issues.

Insusceptible regulating specialists can cause influenza-like side effects, which include:
- Fever
- Chills
- Shortcoming

• Discombobulation
• Nausea or regurgitating
• Muscle or joint throbs
• Exhaustion
• Cerebral pain

Cytokines can likewise cause numerous serious incidental effects namely:
• Inconvenience relaxing
• Low or hypertension
• Extreme unfavorably susceptible responses
• Brought down blood counts, which can raise the gamble of contaminations and cause draining issues
• Blood clusters
• Issues with the state of mind, conduct, thinking, and memory
• Skin issues, for example, rash, consumption at the infusion site, and ulcers
• Organ harm

BCG can likewise cause urinary incidental effects.

Thalidomide, lenalidomide, and pomalidomide can cause:
• Blood clusters
• Nerve issues that lead to torment, deadness, shivering, expanding, or muscle shortcoming in various pieces of the body
• Birth surrenders, whenever utilized during pregnancy

Imiquimod can cause skin responses.

Cancer treated with immunotherapy

Immunotherapy drugs have been supported to treat many kinds of cancer. Be that as it may, immunotherapy isn't yet essentially as generally utilized as surgery, chemotherapy, or radiation treatment.

Symptoms of immunotherapy

Immunotherapy can cause secondary effects, a significant number of which happen when the resistant framework that has been fired up to act against cancer likewise acts against sound cells and tissues in your body.

Side Effects of Immunotherapy

Immunotherapy can cause secondary effects, a significant number of which happen when the resistant framework that has been fired up to act against cancer likewise acts against solid cells and tissues in the body. Various individuals make different side impacts. The ones you have and how they affect you will rely heavily on how solid you are before therapy, your kind of cancer, how cutting-edge it is, the sort of immunotherapy you are getting, and the portion.

You may be on immunotherapy for quite a while, and incidental effects can happen anytime during and after treatment. Specialists and medical attendants can't be aware for certain when or on the other hand on the off chance that incidental effects will happen or how serious they will be. Along these lines, it is essential to understand what signs to search for and what to do on the off chance that you begin to have issues.

A few incidental effects are normal with a wide range of immunotherapy. For example, you could have skin responses at the needle site, which include:

Researching Cancer Immunotherapy Side Effects

Specialists expect to the more likely to comprehend and deal with the symptoms of these new medications.

- Torment
- Expanding
- Irritation
- Redness
- Irritation
- Rash

You might have influenza-like side effects, which include:

- Fever
- Chills
- Shortcoming
- Discombobulation
- Nausea or regurgitating
- Muscle or joint throbs
- Exhaustion
- Cerebral pain
- Inconvenience relaxing
- Low or hypertension

Opposite incidental effects could include:

- Enlarging and weight gain from holding liquid
- Heart palpitations
- Sinus blockage
- Looseness of the bowels
- Contamination
- Organ aggravation

A few kinds of immunotherapy might cause extreme or even deadly unfavorably susceptible and irritation-related responses. Be that as it may, these responses are interesting.

Certain incidental effects could happen relying on the kind of immunotherapy you get. Visit the page for the particular sort of immunotherapy that you are getting for additional insights concerning conceivable serious symptoms of that kind of treatment. These include:

- Insusceptible designated spot inhibitors
- Immune system microorganisms move treatment
- Monoclonal antibodies
- Treatment immunizations
- Insusceptible framework modulators

How is immunotherapy given?

Various types of immunotherapy might be given in various ways. These include:

- Intravenous (IV): The immunotherapy goes straightforwardly into a vein.
- Oral: The immunotherapy comes in pills or containers that you swallow.
- Effective: The immunotherapy arrives in a cream that you rub onto your skin. This sort of immunotherapy can be utilized for early skin cancer.

• Intravesical: The immunotherapy goes straightforwardly into the bladder.

Where do you go for immunotherapy?
You might get immunotherapy in a specialist's office, facility, or short-term unit in an emergency clinic. The short term implies you don't go through the night in the emergency clinic.

How frequently do you get immunotherapy?
How frequently and how lengthy you get immunotherapy relies upon:
• Your sort of cancer and how best in class it is
• The kind of immunotherapy you get
• How your body responds to treatment
You might have treatment consistently, week, or month. A few sorts of immunotherapy are given in cycles. A cycle is a time of treatment followed by a time of rest. The rest time frame allows your body an opportunity to recuperate, answer immunotherapy, and construct new sound cells.

How can you tell if immunotherapy is working?
You will see your primary care physician frequently. The individual in question will give you actual tests and ask you how you feel. You will have clinical trials, for example, blood tests and various kinds of outputs. These tests will quantify the size of your growth and search for changes in your blood work.

Current research in immunotherapy
Specialists are zeroing in on a few significant regions to further develop immunotherapy, including:
• Tracking down answers for obstruction: Specialists are trying blends of insusceptible designated spot inhibitors and different sorts of immunotherapy, designated treatment, and radiation treatment to conquer protection from immunotherapy.
• Tracking down ways of anticipating reactions to immunotherapy: Just a little piece of individuals who get immunotherapy will answer the treatment. Tracking down ways of foreseeing which individuals will answer treatment is a significant area of examination.
• Getting more familiar with how cancer cells sidestep or smother insusceptible reactions against them.
A superior comprehension of how cancer cells get around the insusceptible framework could prompt the improvement of new medications that block those cycles.
• Step-by-step instructions to decrease the symptoms of treatment with immunotherapy.

www.ingramcontent.com/pod-product-compliance
Lightning Source LLC
LaVergne TN
LVHW052100160826
845678LV00015B/3303

* 9 7 9 8 8 4 8 2 4 9 6 1 3 *